THE MINDFUL WAY WORKBOOK

Also from the Authors

For General Readers

The Mindful Way through Depression:
Freeing Yourself from Chronic Unhappiness
Mark Williams, John Teasdale, Zindel Segal,
and Jon Kabat-Zinn

For Professionals

Mindfulness-Based Cognitive Therapy for Depression,
Second Edition
Zindel V. Segal, J. Mark G. Williams,
and John D. Teasdale

Vulnerability to Depression:
From Cognitive Neuroscience to Prevention and Treatment
Rick E. Ingram, Ruth Ann Atchley,
and Zindel V. Segal

For more information, visit *www.mbct.com.*

The Mindful Way
WORKBOOK

AN 8-WEEK PROGRAM TO FREE YOURSELF FROM DEPRESSION AND EMOTIONAL DISTRESS

John Teasdale
Mark Williams
Zindel Segal

Foreword by Jon Kabat-Zinn

THE GUILFORD PRESS
New York   London

For all who seek an end to suffering

© 2014 The Guilford Press
A Division of Guilford Publications, Inc.
370 Seventh Avenue, Suite 1200, New York, NY 10001
www.guilford.com

The information in this volume is not intended as a substitute for consultation with healthcare professionals. Each individual's health concerns should be evaluated by a qualified professional.

Printed in the United States of America

This book is printed on acid-free paper.

Last digit is print number: 9   8   7   6

Library of Congress Cataloging-in-Publication Data
Teasdale, John D.
   The mindful way workbook : an 8-week program to free yourself from depression and emotional distress / John Teasdale, Mark Williams, and Zindel Segal.
      pages cm
   Includes bibliographical references and index.
   ISBN 978-1-4625-0814-3 (pbk.: alk. paper)
   1. Depression, Mental—Treatment.   2. Mindfulness-based cognitive therapy.   3. Meditation—Therapeutic use.   I. Williams, J. Mark G.
II. Segal, Zindel V., 1956–   III. Title.
   RC537.T42   2014
   616.85′27—dc23
                                                                    2013031209

Contents

Purchasers may download audio files and select practical tools
from this book at *www.guilford.com/teasdale-materials.*

Foreword

This book is fantastic. Just how fantastic, it took me a while to realize. I suppose I came to it with a slight prejudice against workbooks in general, and also because I wondered when I first heard that this book was in the works: "Why on earth another book on mindfulness-based cognitive therapy (MBCT), and a workbook at that?" The authors had already done so much to make MBCT accessible to both therapists and the lay public. MBCT has become very popular and highly regarded. People were deriving great benefit from it. What on earth was missing? What more could be said? How much more support for people would be needed? How much more clarity could the authors bring to this subject, and how much more engaging could they possibly make it? It turns out that the answer to all these protestations is: "a lot."

Reading this book and living inside it for a time, I quickly came to see and feel why it is indeed not only necessary but also quite marvelous, and winning. It brings the experience of MBCT and the cultivation of mindfulness to life in a new way, almost as if, in some very real sense, you become a full participant in the program, as if you were *in the classroom*, not only with the instructor but with a whole group of other people whose concerns and questions and—once engaged in the meditation practice—experiences will no doubt very much resemble your own. In this way, I came to see the unique virtues and functions of this workbook form in the skillful hands of the authors. Something was indeed missing in what I had thought was complete.

This book functions as a trusted friend, counselor, and guide, at least as much as a book could possibly manage to do. It gives you, the reader, a sense of being befriended, not so much by the authors personally as by the process itself, as you engage day by day and week by week in this simple yet potentially profoundly liberating exploration of your own mind and body through the cultivation of mindfulness. It walks us through a process that illuminates the ways in which old habits of mind can so easily imprison us, even though at face value our thoughts are in the service of trying to make sense of things and improve our lot.

One of the most endearing and useful features of this book are the balloons that speak back and forth, posing the questions we might be thinking or pondering ourselves, and then offering answers that might help us see things in new ways, in more kind and freeing ways. Here are the voices of the other people in your class, practicing in parallel with you, asking questions and reporting on their experiences, just as you might. And here are the gentle, extremely clear, and highly reassuring responses of the instructor to the various questions and uncertainties that arise every day about how to practice, what to practice, and whether you are "doing it right," in other words, whether what you are experiencing is valid. And the gentle and reassuring voice is always here, reminding you over and over again that what you are experiencing *is* valid because it is your experience, and because you are aware of it.

This is the growing edge of learning from your own experience, of learning by trusting your own experience when it is held in awareness—of seeing through and going beyond the usual frames of good and bad, liking and disliking, and finding new ways of *being in relationship* to what might previously have driven you mad, or into distress of some kind, into a downward spiral of endless and unhelpful rumination and darkness. Engaging fully in the program offered here teaches you to invite such moments back into the family of the living and of your own life, and that while it takes bravery to do it, the benefits are enormous. It shows you with great clarity and compassion that what you might previously have thought of as your fate is no longer your fate, and never was—that you, like all of us, are presented with endless opportunities to exercise your muscles of learning, growing, and healing once you know this is possible, and thereby transform your life; that you, like all of us, are presented with endless opportunities for realizing that you have very real choices, moment by moment, regarding how you will be in relationship to what is unfolding in your own mind, in your own body, and in the world.

It turns out that this simple shift in perspective moment by moment—especially in those moments that are tough, or frightening, or discouraging—makes all the difference. It can give your life back to you, in all its fullness and beauty. I hope it does. Living inside this book and engaging wholeheartedly in the curriculum it offers—where whatever arises in your life and in your mind becomes an essential part of that curriculum—can make all the difference. May you inhabit this new way of being as best you can, moment by moment, and let your doing flow out of your being. May you practice hard, may you practice gently, and with kindness. You are in good hands here, including, and especially, your own.

JON KABAT-ZINN
Lexington, Massachusetts
April 22, 2013

Acknowledgments

Over the years, many people have contributed generously to the development, dissemination, and evaluation of mindfulness-based cognitive therapy (MBCT). Here we offer our acknowledgments and thanks specifically to those who have contributed to the process of creating this workbook.

From its inception, this project has been steered skillfully forward by Kitty Moore, Senior Editor at The Guilford Press. We have been wonderfully fortunate in once more enjoying the benefits of the creative talents, sensitive encouragement, and wise editorial guidance of Chris Benton. David Moore produced the attractive and clear figures, responding promptly to each nuanced change we asked of him. Kevin Porter, from A Musik Zone, and Heavy Entertainment (*www.heavy-entertainment.com*) were the sound engineers for the audio tracks. We greatly appreciate the help of all these individuals and thank them warmly.

We acknowledge with great gratitude the input of Trish Bartley, Melanie Fennell, Jackie Teasdale, and Phyllis Williams, who put aside other commitments to read a late draft of the manuscript on very short notice. Their feedback transformed both the appearance and tone of the book.

It is a great delight to acknowledge the foundational, inspirational, collegial, and substantive contributions of Jon Kabat-Zinn to the development of MBCT. Our collaboration has been a continuing source of joy and learning. We offer him our wholehearted thanks for graciously agreeing to write the foreword to this book.

Finally, it is a pleasure to have this opportunity to express our deep appreciation to the participants in mindfulness-based programs we have offered. Their contributions have profoundly shaped the development of MBCT and the substance of this book. Some have generously given us their stories; others were the inspiration for the interactions we illustrate; all were our teachers. We thank them, every one.

Publishers and authors have generously given permission to reprint material from the following copyrighted works:

"How Does Mindfulness Transform Suffering? I: The Nature and Origins of *Dukkha*," by John D. Teasdale and Michael Chaskalson. In *Contemporary Buddhism: An Interdisciplinary Journal*, 2011, *12* (1), 89–102. Copyright 2011 by Taylor & Francis. Reprinted by permission of Taylor & Francis Ltd.

The Mindful Way through Depression, by Mark Williams, John Teasdale, Zindel Segal, and Jon Kabat-Zinn. Copyright 2007 by The Guilford Press. Adapted by permission.

Mindfulness-Based Cognitive Therapy for Depression, Second Edition, by Zindel V. Segal, J. Mark G. Williams, and John D. Teasdale. Copyright 2013 by The Guilford Press. Adapted and reprinted by permission.

The Way It Is: New and Selected Poems, by William E. Stafford. Copyright 1998 by the Estate of William Stafford. Reprinted by permission of The Permissions Company on behalf of Graywolf Press.

"Dreaming the Real," by Linda France. In Abhinando Bhikkhu (Ed.), *Tomorrow's Moon.* Copyright 2005 by Linda France. Reprinted by permission.

New Collected Poems, by Wendell Berry. Copyright 2012 by Wendell Berry. Reprinted by permission of Counterpoint.

"Cognitive Self-Statements in Depression: Development of an Automatic Thoughts Questionnaire," by Steven D. Hollon and Philip C. Kendall. In *Cognitive Therapy and Research,* 1980, *4,* 383–395. Copyright 1980 by Philip C. Kendall and Steven D. Hollon. Adapted by permission of the authors.

Dream Work, by Mary Oliver. Copyright 1986 by Mary Oliver. Reprinted by permission of Grove/Atlantic.

The Essential Rumi, by Coleman Barks and John Moyne. Copyright 1995 by Coleman Barks and John Moyne. Reprinted by permission of Threshold Books.

The Dance, by Oriah Mountain Dreamer. Copyright 2001 by Oriah Mountain Dreamer. Reprinted by permission of HarperCollins Publishers.

Insight Meditation: The Practice of Freedom, by Joseph Goldstein. Copyright 1994 by Joseph Goldstein. Reprinted by permission of Shambhala Publications.

Full Catastrophe Living, by Jon Kabat-Zinn. Copyright 1990 by Jon Kabat-Zinn. Adapted by permission of Dell Publishing, a division of Random House.

House of Light, by Mary Oliver. Copyright 1990 by Mary Oliver. Reprinted by permission of The Charlotte Sheedy Literary Agency.

Some Tips for Everyday Mindfulness, by Madeline Klyne, Executive Director, Cambridge Insight Meditation Center. Copyright by Madeline Klyne. Adapted by permission of the author.

Collected Poems, 1948–1984, by Derek Walcott. Copyright 1986 by Derek Walcott. Reprinted by permission of Farrar, Straus and Giroux and Faber and Faber.

Authors' Note

Participant Quotations

Throughout the book we give quotations from previous participants in MBCT programs. Some of these are close to verbatim quotations from specific participants. Where they have suggested using their own first names we have done so; otherwise, we have given participants aliases. In other cases, the statements represent the essence of quotations from a number of participants, and the identities are purely fictional. We also include many examples of interactions between participants and instructors—again, these represent typical recurring exchanges, rather than the actual words of specific individuals.

Notes

At the end of the book, the Notes section provides references for some of the assertions we make, the sources of poems and other quotations from books, and acknowledgments for the permission to reproduce material.

Audio Files

A list of the audio tracks included on the MP3 CD that accompanies this book is given on page 228. The tracks are also available to download from The Guilford Press website, *www.guilford.com/teasdale-materials*.

You can listen to the MP3 CD in many ways. If you have an MP3-enabled CD player (look for an MP3 logo on the device), you can play this disc just like any audio CD. You can play it on most computers by simply inserting it into the CD tray. You can also then copy the files onto an MP3 player or import the files into your iTunes library and listen on the go.

Part I

Foundations

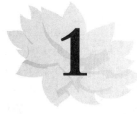

Welcome

Welcome to the 8-week MBCT program. MBCT stands for mindfulness-based cognitive therapy. It is a program specifically designed to help you deal with persistent unwanted mood states.

MBCT has been tested in research and proven effective for depression, as well as for anxiety and a wide range of other problems.

You can use this book in a number of ways: as a member of a professionally guided MBCT class, as part of individual therapy, or as self-help.

We wish you well as you embark on this voyage—to discover how you may best nourish your deepest capacity for wholeness and healing.

If you've ever been deeply unhappy with your life for any length of time, you know how difficult it can be to do anything about it. No matter how hard you may try, things just don't get better—or not for long. You feel stressed out, exhausted with the effort of just keeping going. Life has lost its color, and you don't seem to know how to get it back.

Gradually you may come to believe that there must be something wrong with *you,* that fundamentally you are just not good enough.

This sense of inner emptiness might come from an accumulation of stresses over a long period of time or from one or two traumatic events that unexpectedly dislocate your life. It might even just arise out of the blue without any apparent cause. You might find yourself lost in inconsolable sorrow; feeling profoundly empty; or painfully disappointed with yourself, with other people, or with the world in general.

For anyone who experiences emotional problems that won't go away, the despair and demoralization, the sheer joylessness of depression, is never very far away.

If these feelings escalate, they may become severe enough to be called clinical depression. But the sort of unhappiness we are speaking of here touches all of us from time to time.

For any of us who find ourselves with low mood of any magnitude or duration—whether it's major depression; persistent, nagging unhappiness; or intermittent periods of the blues that feel disruptive or disabling—the despair and demoralization, the sheer joylessness typical of depression, are never very far away.

When things get overwhelming, we may distract ourselves for a while, but questions keep nagging at the back of the mind: "Why can't I pull myself out of this?" "What if it stays this way forever?" "What's wrong with me?"

Bringing Back Hope

What if, despite what your thoughts may try to tell you, there is nothing wrong with *you* at all?

What if your heroic efforts to prevent your feelings from getting the best of you are actually backfiring?

What if they are the very things that are keeping you stuck in suffering or even making things worse?

This book is written to help you understand how this happens and what you can do about it.

Mindfulness-Based Cognitive Therapy (MBCT)

In these pages we will guide you, step by step, through the MBCT program.

This research-based 8-week course is designed to give you the skills and understanding that will empower you to free yourself from getting entangled in painful emotions.

MBCT Is Effective

All over the world, research has shown MBCT can halve the risk of future clinical depression in people who have already been depressed several times—its effects seem just as good as antidepressant medications.

Of course, depression often arrives hand in hand with anxiety, irritability, or other unwanted emotions. The good news is that while MBCT was developed and has proven extremely effective for depression, research is now also showing powerful effects of MBCT on persistent anxiety and other destructive emotions.

The heart of MBCT is gentle, systematic training in mindfulness (we'll say more about what mindfulness is later).

This training frees us from the grip of two critical processes that lie at the root of depression and many other emotional problems:

1. the tendency to overthink, ruminate, or worry too much about some things,

   coupled with

2. a tendency to avoid, suppress, or push away other things.

If you have suffered long-term emotional difficulties, you'll have already discovered that worrying or suppressing doesn't really help.

But you may feel powerless to stop it.

Redoubling your efforts to switch off your troubled mind may give temporary relief, but it can also make things worse.

Your attention is still hijacked by whatever is troubling you: it's so difficult to prevent the mind from being dragged back again and again to the very place from which you want to escape.

What if it were possible to learn wholly new skills that allowed you to cultivate a radically different way of working with your mind?

> **Jessica:** *"My problem was always lying awake at night brooding about what had happened at work during the day and worrying about what was going to happen tomorrow. I tried everything to try to stop my thoughts, but nothing worked. It just got worse. Then this [the brooding] started happening during the day as well. I was even forgetting what I was supposed to be doing. That's when I realized things had gone past the point where I could help myself."*

Mindfulness training teaches exactly these skills: it gives you back control of your attention so that, moment by moment, you can experience yourself and the world without the harsh self-critical voice of judgment that may so often follow you around.

Daily practice of mindfulness reduces the tendency to brood and worry about everything.

You wake up to the small beauties and pleasures of the world.

You learn to respond wisely and compassionately to the people and events that affect you.

We developed MBCT, and we have seen, over and over again, how it liberates people

> **Mindfulness** means being able to bring direct, open-hearted awareness to what you are doing while you are doing it: being able to tune in to what's going on in your mind and body, and in the outside world, moment by moment.

from their burden of low mood and the stress and exhaustion that goes with it. We've seen the extraordinary consequences of their discovery that there is a way to live life more fully than they ever imagined.

> "My son said the other day 'You're in such a good mood these days'—and I felt a smile inside myself, and I gave him a hug."

> "I started reaching out to friends to get together more often—I'd been afraid to do that—and now my phone rings more often—friends calling with ideas for going out."

> "Before I came here, I didn't know what it was like to live without pressure. I might have had some idea when I was 5 years old, but I can't remember much of that. I have been shown a different way to live, and it's so simple."

> "I started painting again for the first time since I was in college."

> "My daughter says my posture and my walk are entirely different—and I realized she was right . . . I feel lighter somehow."

Who Is This Book For?

This book is for anyone who wishes to take the 8-week MBCT program.

This might be as part of a class taught by an instructor, as part of individual therapy, or as a form of self-help, working through the program by yourself or with a friend. Whichever of these routes you take, you will be supported on a daily basis by the guided practices recorded on the CD or audio downloads that come with the book.

And, of course, you don't have to have been seriously depressed to find the MBCT program valuable:

- Research is constantly expanding the range of emotional problems that benefit from MBCT.
- MBCT focuses on the core psychological processes that lie at the root of many different ways in which we can get stuck in unhappiness.

> ### What If You Are Very Depressed Right Now?
>
> MBCT was originally designed to help people who had previously suffered serious depressions. It was offered to them at a time when they were relatively well, as a way to learn skills to prevent depression from coming back. There is overwhelming evidence that the program is effective in doing that.
>
> There is also growing evidence that MBCT can help people while they are in the midst of a depression.
>
> But if things are really bad right now, and your depression makes it just too difficult to concentrate on some of the practices, then it can be disheartening to struggle with new learning. It might be most skillful to allow yourself to wait a while if you can, or, if you do start, to be very gentle with yourself—remembering that the difficulties you experience are a direct effect of depression and will, sooner or later, ease.

The patterns of mind that keep people trapped in emotional suffering are fundamentally the same patterns of mind that stand between all of us and the flowering of our potential for a more deeply satisfying way of being.

Why Another Book?

We have already written one book describing MBCT for a wide audience: *The Mindful Way through Depression* (coauthored with our colleague Jon Kabat-Zinn, the principal figure catalyzing and guiding the surge of interest in mindfulness that has swept the world in recent decades).

That book and this workbook complement each other; it is very helpful to use them in tandem.

If you have not read *The Mindful Way through Depression*, you may find it a useful general introduction to the MBCT approach. It gives a lot of background detail that might be particularly helpful if you are using this workbook on your own, as self-help.

If you have already read *The Mindful Way through Depression*, this workbook will give you all the additional tools and detailed practical guidance you need to take yourself through the MBCT program.

Why a Workbook?

The form of this book is specifically designed to support and guide you through a program that can lead to radical and lasting changes in your life and well-being.

It is rare for such changes to come about just by **reading about** how we get entangled in emotional turmoil and what we can do to free ourselves.

Rather, profound and lasting change usually involves taking some kind of **action**—what, in this book, we call **practice.** It is in this work, done day by day, that 99 percent of the learning in MBCT goes on.

Inner transformation depends on a continuing back-and-forth dance between understanding, practice, and reflection. The new insights and skills that emerge are **embodied** deep in our being—that is why they can have such widespread and enduring effects.

This workbook provides three elements, crucial to this dance of transformation: a STRUCTURE, a chance for REFLECTION, and a source of INSIGHT.

The **structure** means that you have in your hand a map that will guide you day by day along the path of change. The itinerary for each day's journey is spelled out in detail. Once you have made an initial commitment to follow the path, you can simply relax into what is there to be done for that day, for that moment.

Space for short **reflections** is built into the fabric of the book. These give you the chance to pause, to stand back, and to see more clearly what is going on in mind and body and in the world around you. From such reflections insights arise.

The book further supports the development of **insight** by offering, after each practice or exercise, a dialogue reflecting aspects of what other participants discover during the practice. Reading these will help you make sense of what has been happening for you too. In moving in close to your own experience in this way, you begin to make your own discoveries—and gain insight into the possibilities of a greater freedom and well-being.

For many people, the most helpful approach might be to read *The Mindful Way through Depression* (or have it available for reference) along with using this workbook. Many find it most effective to do this in the company of others, working through MBCT in a group with a trained teacher.

The Shape of the Book

In Chapters 2 and 3 we consider the essential questions: Why do we find ourselves, time after time, sinking into depression or getting stuck in emotional distress? How do the practices and exercises of the 8-week MBCT program make a difference? How might all this help you?

With this understanding in place, Chapter 4 looks at how best to prepare for the course. Then, in the following seven chapters, we move, step by step, week by week, through the nuts and bolts of the program.

Finally, in the concluding chapter of the book we look to the future. We consider how, if you wish, you might further nourish and extend the ways in which mindfulness can transform and enrich your life.

> "Since doing the program I have been able to actually enjoy and be in the present moment . . . realizing this is the only time I have to live . . . so instead of constantly worrying about the future and my past failures, I can more evenly embrace the present moment.
>
> "It's not exaggerating to say that MBCT has changed me in just about every way possible."

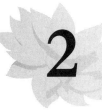

2

Depression, Unhappiness, and Emotional Distress

WHY DO WE GET STUCK?

Jani would often wake very early in the morning, unable to sleep, with a heavy feeling in her body and thoughts going round and round, impossible to switch off. She'd sometimes get up to make a cup of tea, sitting in the kitchen with a blanket around her shoulders, reading bits of any magazine that she or her roommate had left lying around, or opening her laptop and trying to answer e-mails that had come in overnight. At last, exhausted, she'd go back to bed, only to find that the thoughts carried on, going round and round, but now with a new voice: "This is terrible. You'll be too tired to think straight today. Why is this happening again? Why can't you ever pull yourself together? What's wrong with you?"

For any of us it would be bad enough to wake up too early in this way. But Jani's mind just made things worse.

Reading through the story again, can you now see any similarities between the ways in which the "new voice" added its own twist to Jani's misery and your own past experience?

Put a ✔ next to any of these that you recognize:

☐ The voice added its own catastrophic interpretation ("This is terrible") to the situation.

☐ The voice was certain there would be awful consequences ("You'll be too tired to think straight").

The voice asked unanswerable questions that had the effect of:

☐ bringing to mind times in the past when things had gone wrong ("Why is this happening again? Why can't you ever pull yourself together?")

☐ focusing attention on weaknesses and failings ("What's wrong with you?")

Jani's experience illustrates a crucial and unexpected truth:

Unhappiness Itself Is Not the Problem

Unhappiness is part of the normal human condition. It is a natural response to certain situations. Left to itself, it will pass in its own good time, often surprisingly quickly.

But, somehow, most of us don't feel able to let things take their natural course—when we feel sad or unhappy, we feel **we have to *do* something**, even if it's only trying to understand what's going on.

Paola: *"I find I can't leave it alone once I get these moods. I sort of know it doesn't do me any good to worry and brood, but I can't help it."*

Paradoxically, it is those very attempts to get rid of unwanted unhappy feelings that get us stuck in ever-deepening unhappiness.

> Our reactions to unhappiness can transform what might otherwise be a brief, passing sadness into persistent dissatisfaction and unhappiness.

Let's look more closely at what's going on here.
We can distinguish three crucial stages:

Stage 1: Unhappiness arises.

Stage 2: The unhappy mood brings up negative thinking patterns, feelings, and memories from the past—this makes us more unhappy.

Stage 3: We try to get rid of the unhappiness in ways that actually keep it going and just make things worse.

The Echoes of the Past

A few years ago Jani had been totally stressed by the amount of work she was expected to do in the job she held at the time. She'd become very down and constantly tried to "pull herself together" before eventually going to her physician, who prescribed antidepressant medication, which helped a bit.

She'd eventually left that job, but somehow she still blamed herself for giving in. Now, 7 years later in the early hours, as she struggled with not being able to sleep but not being really awake either, thinking of the day ahead, this echo of the past was making her feel worse.

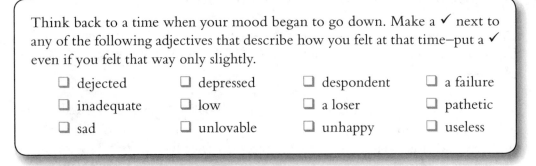

Think back to a time when your mood began to go down. Make a ✔ next to any of the following adjectives that describe how you felt at that time—put a ✔ even if you felt that way only slightly.

- ❏ dejected
- ❏ depressed
- ❏ despondent
- ❏ a failure
- ❏ inadequate
- ❏ low
- ❏ a loser
- ❏ pathetic
- ❏ sad
- ❏ unlovable
- ❏ unhappy
- ❏ useless

There are actually two different kinds of words in this list. Some are simply descriptions of moods or feelings (*dejected, depressed, despondent, low, sad, unhappy*). The others describe feelings that also seem to say something about the kind of person you are (*a failure, inadequate, a loser, pathetic, unlovable, useless*).

> If you have been depressed in the past, thoughts of self-criticism or of being a failure are much more likely to get switched on by sad moods.

Research using this list of words has revealed something very important.

If you have been seriously depressed in the past, when you start to feel low now—*whatever the reason*—you are much more likely to begin to feel bad about yourself (and so check off words like *a failure*) than someone who has never been so depressed.

This is because, whenever we are very down, the mind is taken over by patterns of extremely negative thinking—thoughts that we are worthless, thoughts that we have let people down, thoughts that life is full of insurmountable difficulties, thoughts that the future is hopeless.

> **Bill:** *"Basically, I feel that I am just not good enough—and sooner or later people will find out."*

Links get forged between these thinking patterns and depressed, unhappy mood.

The result? Sad mood arises now and old negative thinking patterns are right behind.

Tragically, these are exactly the feelings and thought patterns that would make anyone even more depressed.

And so the cycle continues: if you have been deeply depressed, it is much easier to slide back into depression again.

It's not only thinking patterns that can get reawakened. Spells of depression will have often been triggered by experiences of major loss, rejection, or failure.

Anna: *"Here I go again. I just feel like I have no future; that nothing has worked for me in the past and nothing will change. I can't stand much more of this."*

When you feel sad or depressed again, memories of these losses and rejections—and all the weight of their tragedy—can break over you like a tidal wave. In that way, these thoughts and memories will make you even sadder, adding their own twist to a spiral of worsening mood.

For Jani, her frustration with not getting to sleep and her fears about not being able to cope with her job evoked memories that made her feel even worse:

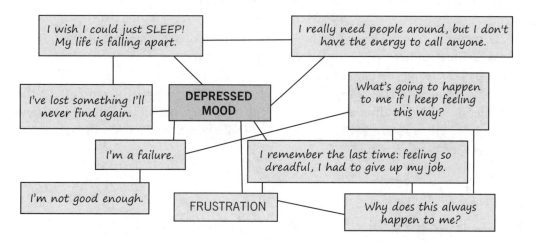

Just like Jani's depression, other emotions can color our experience in subtle (and not-so-subtle) ways, with consequences we cannot always see clearly.

For example:

- Feelings of anxiety can reawaken worrisome patterns of thinking— creating more anxiety, worries, and fears.

Moods and feelings can trigger "matching" patterns of thinking, memory, and attention, which then make the feelings even more intense and persistent.

Olga: *"What will happen if Bob gets ill again? Will I be able to cope? I don't want to be alone."*

- Feelings of irritation and frustration can make us blame and criticize others, making us even more angry and frustrated.

> **Scott:** "G. had no right to do this. If he does this again, it will be the last straw. I'm supposed to be responsible for running this project, not him."

- If we are overstressed by excessive demands, feelings of pressure may reawaken fears of being overwhelmed and force us to greater busyness and stress.

> **Pearl:** "No one else can do this. It's all up to me. This deadline is really important."

The good news is that, with the right understanding and skills, we can break out of these mood–thought vicious cycles.

Over and over, we have seen people learn to recognize these thought patterns for what they really are—just thought patterns—and then gracefully disengage from them by refocusing their attention.

The problem is that, through no fault of our own, most of us don't have the appropriate understanding and skills. In fact, you may have found that your best-intentioned efforts often have exactly the opposite effect to what you intended.

Let's see how.

How Trying to Dig Your Way Out of Trouble Can End Up Digging You In Deeper

> **Carmen:** "If I don't snap out of this soon, I'll be over the edge again. I've got to do something."

> **Tony:** "I had such plans when I was young. Where did it all go? How did I end up like this? What is it about me? What's wrong with me?"

If you have experienced low mood spiraling down to deeper depression in the past, you will know just how horrible that can be. It's completely understandable to feel the urge to get rid of the mood and stop the slide into something deeper.

Equally, if feeling constantly exhausted and unable to enjoy life reawakens a deep doubt about your worth as a person, what could feel more important than doing something about that?

If we look carefully, we can see what is happening here:

The mind is trying to get rid of unhappiness by thinking its way out of the problem.

> Think back once more to a time when your mood started to go down. Did any thoughts like these go through your mind?
>
> "What's wrong with me that I get so unhappy when other people seem to have friends and be happy?"
>
> "What did I do wrong to end up feeling like this?"
>
> "What's going to happen to me if I keep feeling this way?"

These kinds of questions have no clear answer. Nonetheless, we feel compelled to keep chewing away at them—a process that psychologists call rumination.

Psychologist Susan Nolen-Hoeksema spent many years investigating rumination and its effects. Her conclusions are stark:

Ruminating just makes us feel even worse:

We suffer the frustration of not being able to come up with answers.

We dredge up memories of failures and difficulties from the past to try to understand how we get things wrong. But focusing on our weaknesses and deficiencies in this way only drags us down further.

We anticipate the problems that will arise in the future if things don't change and dread the prospect of having to face the days, weeks, and months ahead.

We may even begin to wonder whether life is worth living at all.

Far from freeing us from the downward spiral, **our attempts to get rid of unhappiness by thinking our way out of it are the very things that can deepen and prolong our sad moods**. These moods then bring up more unhappy memories and thoughts, and we now have new material to ruminate on.

If you have been clinically depressed in the past, rumination can create a slide in mood that will tip you into another episode of depression.

Asha: *"All this thinking is getting me nowhere."*

Phil: *"It's always been this way. I'm sure I've lost friends by being so negative. What makes me do this? I remember the time when . . ."*

Diana: *"Something in my life has been damaged forever."*

> The problem with persistent and recurrent depression, unhappiness, and exhaustion is not "feeling low" in the first place. The problem is what happens next.
>
> **The core problem is how our minds react to feeling low, afraid, angry, or tired.**

Why Do We Get Locked in a Struggle We Can't Win?

Rumination can cause us enormous difficulties. It can transform the simple experience of a fleeting emotion of sadness into serious depression; a fleeting emotion of irritation into a prolonged sense of indignation and anger; a fleeting moment of concern into a deep sense of anxiety.

So why do we do it? Why do we ruminate, brood, and worry, when, far from rescuing us from destructive emotions, this actually makes things worse?

To answer these questions, and to help us understand how we might begin to respond differently, let's step back and look briefly at the way the mind works more generally.

The Doing Mode of Mind

To solve a problem or to get things done, the mind usually works in certain predictable ways.

Take, for example, a day when you have to take a detour from your usual drive home to drop off a package at a friend's house, but you find yourself driving past the point where you meant to turn off into his or her street.

After a few moments, you notice the package is still there and realize that this is not what you had intended. You think **back**: "Ah, I should have taken the other turn." You think **forward**: "What shall I do next?"

You work out that the simplest way to sort things out is to turn around and make a deliberate effort, this time, to (1) turn off at the exit to your friend's house and (2) not just drive straight past it, as you normally would.

You act on these plans, take the right route, and deliver the package to your friend—mission accomplished!

The package eventually arrived at its destination through your mind's use of a very well-rehearsed and familiar mental routine.

This routine helps us get things done—achieve goals, solve problems, change things to make them more like we want them to be.

We call this the **"doing" mode of mind.** You'll find its core features listed in the box below.

To work effectively, at each point the doing mode has to *hold in mind*, and then *compare*, three ideas:

1. where you are at each moment (the **current state**)

2. where you want to be (your destination, **goal**, or **desired outcome**)

3. where you don't want to be (your nondestination or **outcome you want to avoid**)

By holding and comparing these three ideas the mind can see how well the current state of affairs matches up with the goal you want to achieve and is different from the outcome you want to avoid.

Knowing whether these gaps are increasing or decreasing allows the doing mode to "steer" the mind and body in the right direction and reach the desired goal and/or avoid the undesired destination.

We are not necessarily conscious of all these processes. Many of them are carried out automatically in the background of awareness.

By using the same "doing" strategy the human mind can achieve some remarkable goals—from developing computers to building cities and putting a man on the moon.

Seven Core Features of the Doing Mode

1. It often comes on line **automatically.**

2. It uses **thoughts and ideas**, holding them in mind as you work.

3. It **dwells in the past and future** to help get where you want to be.

4. It keeps in mind what to **avoid**—where you **don't** want to end up.

5. It **needs things to be different**, forever focusing on the gap between where you are and where you want to be.

6. It takes **thoughts/ideas as real** (it would not be useful to keep doubting your destination).

7. Left to itself, it **continues to focus on the goal** until the task is complete, or until you are too tired and depleted to continue. The demands of the doing mode can be quite **harsh** and **unkind.**

If Doing Is So Useful, What Goes Wrong?

If we want to achieve goals by making changes in the world around us—like building a house—the doing mode of mind is brilliantly effective.

So, it makes sense that the mind turns to the same basic strategy when we want to achieve goals in our inner, personal worlds—goals like feeling happy, not feeling anxious, being a spontaneous person, or not being someone who gets depressed.

It is here that things can go horribly wrong.

For now there is a major difference. To solve problems, the doing mode has to hold in mind the ideas of where we are, where we want to be, and where we don't want to be. To work at all, these have to be held at the back of the mind all the time until the problem is solved or let go of.

For *external* problems like driving to a destination, holding these ideas in mind does not itself affect the distance left to travel.

But what about those times when the goal is *internal*—to be happy, or *not* to have certain unwanted feelings, or *not* to be a certain kind of person?

Remember how the doing mode works. Now we have to hold in mind "I'm unhappy"; "I wish I were happier"; "I don't want these horrible feelings to come back." What happens now?

Try saying these sentences to yourself two or three times:

"I'm unhappy."

"I wish I were happier."

"I don't want these horrible feelings to come back."

The doing mode needs to keep in mind the gap between the kind of person we are and the kind of person we want to be. But this just reminds us how much we are falling short of where we feel we need to be, creating more unhappiness.

What was your experience? You probably felt worse. Most people do.

The gap between where you are now and where you want to be just got **bigger**.

It is not just the ideas held in the mind that cause problems; it is **comparing** them.

Sometimes the mind can see what's going on and just let go of the project to get rid of unwanted feelings altogether.

At other times the mind feels compelled to continue: if we've known many times when sadness has led to depression, there will be an understandable *fear* of unhappiness—we'll feel a need to avoid experiencing unhappiness at all costs.

That way, we believe, we'll prevent ourselves from slipping back yet again into the depths of emotional turmoil. Here the mind just cannot let go—it will feel like we need *at all costs* to get rid of the negative feelings.

This is where the doing mode becomes the **"driven–doing"** mode:

Driven–doing is the mode of mind where we feel
we just cannot let go of trying to get what we want
or get rid of what we don't want.

Ruminative worry is just one form of driven–doing—the mind *redoubling its efforts* to apply the power of the doing mode to a problem to which it is tragically unsuited.

Rumination turns to the doing mode to "fix" sadness and unhappiness because this pattern of mind really does work very well when we have to get things done in the external world.

But when it comes to fixing what is going on in our internal worlds, in what we see as "me," rumination and doing backfire disastrously.

So what can we do instead?

There are two key steps to responding more skillfully:

1. Learning to recognize ruminative worry and driven–doing as they arise in our moment-by-moment experience and to see them for what they are.

2. Cultivating an alternative mode of mind that allows us to respond more skillfully to sadness, unhappiness, and other unpleasant emotions and unwanted inner experiences.

In Chapter 3 we will introduce that alternative mode and describe where and how mindfulness fits into the overall scheme of things.

Doing, Being, and Mindfulness

Doing is just one of a number of different modes in which the mind can work.

We can think of these different modes as somewhat like the different gears of a car, each mode of mind serving a different function or purpose.

And, just as a car can be in only one gear at a time, so the mind can be in only one mode at a time.

This is really important—it means **we can free ourselves from any problems the doing mode creates by moving into another, different mode**—we can learn how "to shift mental gears."

Design a Different Mode of Mind

On the facing page we summarize the seven core features of the doing mind introduced in Chapter 2. Next to each feature is a space for you to write a word or two to describe what the opposite of that feature would look like. The first one has been written in as an example. What would a good alternative to the doing mode look like?

**The Seven Core Features
of the Doing Mode**

Possible alternative:

1. Often automatic

1. *deliberate, on purpose*

2. Works through thinking

2. _____

3. Focuses on past and future

3. _____

4. Tries to avoid unpleasant experiences

4. _____

5. Needs things to be different

5. _____

6. Takes thoughts/ideas as real

6. _____

7. Focuses on what needs to be done, ignoring undesirable side effects, such as being unkind to oneself or others

7. _____

Being and Doing

Good news! We **already have** a wonderful alternative to the doing mode of mind. It is the mode of **being.** It is a mode with which most of us are not very familiar, but the exercise you just did may have given you clues as to what being looks like.

In the next few pages, we describe the being mode by contrasting it, feature by feature, with the seven core features of the doing mode.

A central aim of the MBCT program is to learn how to recognize these two modes in your own life so that you know when to switch from doing to being.

As a first step, we invite you to estimate, feature by feature, the balance between doing and being in your own everyday experience. Please circle the appropriate phrase after each pair of boxes to indicate your estimate.

1. Living on "Automatic Pilot" versus Living with Conscious Awareness and Choice

IN DOING MODE we live on automatic pilot much of the time: we drive, walk, eat, even speak without clear awareness of what we are doing. Doing starts up automatically whenever there is a mismatch between where we are now and where we want to be. Focusing narrowly on our goals, we rarely stop and notice the wonder of what is happening around us as we move through our lives. We can end up missing much of our lives, forever postponing the time when life will be less hectic and we'll really notice things again.	THE BEING MODE *is intentional rather than automatic. This means we can choose what to do next, rather than run on old, worn-out habits. This allows us to see things as if for the very first time. We "reinhabit" the present moment and become fully conscious of our lives. Being brings a freshness to our perception. We become fully alive and aware again.*

Based on this feature, which of the following best describes the balance between doing and being in your life from day to day? (Circle one.)

More doing than being	Equal doing and being	More being than doing

2. Relating to Experience through Thought versus Directly Sensing Experience

THE DOING MODE works on *ideas*—that's what goals are. It thinks *about* the world in which we dwell, *about* the kind of person we are, *about* the feelings, sensations, and thoughts we have—thinking, thinking, thinking fills our minds much of the time. When we deal with a thought about life as if it were the "real thing," we live one step back from life—we connect with life indirectly through a veil of thoughts that filters out the color, vibrancy, and energy of life.	IN BEING MODE *we connect with life directly—we sense it, we experience it, we know it intimately by close acquaintance. We get a taste of the richness and ever-shifting wonder of the experience of life.*

For this feature, estimate the balance of doing and being in your life (circle one):

More doing than being	Equal doing and being	More being than doing

3. Dwelling on and in the Past and Future versus Being Fully in the Present Moment

IN DOING, we engage in mental time travel. Our minds go forward to the future—to our ideas of how we want things to be—or back to the past, to memories of similar situations, to see what guidance they can offer. In mental time travel we feel as though we are actually *in* the future or *in* the past. This disconnects us from experiencing the fullness of life in the present. We can easily wind up ruminating on the past, re-experiencing the pain of past losses and failures. Worrying about the future, we experience fear and anxiety over threats and dangers that may never happen.	IN BEING, *the mind is gathered, here, now, in this moment, fully present and available to whatever the universe may offer. We can have thoughts about the future and memories of the past—but, crucially, we experience them as parts of our* present *experience. We witness them without being drawn into the past or future worlds the thoughts might otherwise create.*

For this feature, estimate the balance of doing and being in your life (circle one):

More doing than being	Equal doing and being	More being than doing

4. Needing to Avoid, Escape, or Get Rid of Unpleasant Experience versus Approaching It with Interest

IN DOING MODE the immediate, automatic reaction to any unpleasant experience is to set up a goal—to avoid the experience, to push it away, to get rid of it, or to destroy it. This reaction is called **aversion**. Aversion underlies all the thinking patterns that get us stuck in unwanted emotions.	IN BEING, *the basic response is to* **approach** *all experience, even the unpleasant, with interest and respect.* *There is no setting of goals for how things should be or should not be. Rather, there is a natural interest and curiosity in all* experience—*whether it is pleasant, unpleasant, or neither.*

For this feature, estimate the balance of doing and being in your life (circle one):

More doing than being	Equal doing and being	More being than doing

5. Needing Things to Be Different versus Allowing Things to Be Just as They Already Are

DOING is dedicated to **change**—to making things more like we think they should be, less like we think they shouldn't be. Always **focusing on the gap** between what is and what should be, we can have an underlying sense that we or our experiences are falling short in some way—we or they are just "not good enough." This sense of unsatisfactoriness can quite easily turn into self-criticism and self-judgment. There is a basic lack of kindness to ourselves and our experience.	BEING *brings with it an underlying attitude of "allowing" to ourselves and to our experience. There is no demand that experience fit in with our ideas of how it should be—being allows experience to be just as it already is. We can be content with experience, even if it feels unpleasant. We can be content with ourselves, even if, from the perspective of the doing mode, we are not all we should be. This radical acceptance embodies a basic attitude of unconditional kindness and goodwill.*

For this feature, estimate the balance of doing and being in your life (circle one):

More doing than being	Equal doing and being	More being than doing

6. Seeing Thoughts as True and Real versus Seeing Them as Mental Events

DOING MODE treats thoughts and ideas about things as if they were the same as the things themselves. But **the thought of a meal is not the meal itself**—a thought is just a mental event—very, very different from the reality of the experience it is about. If we forget this and treat thoughts as reality, then when we think "I'm a failure," we can feel as if we had just *experienced* being a failure.	IN BEING, *we experience thoughts as part of the flow of life—in just the same way we experience sensations, sounds, feelings, and sights. We cultivate the ability to experience thoughts **as thoughts**—as mental events that enter and leave the mind. With this shift, we rob thoughts of their power to upset us or to control our actions. When we see thoughts for what they are—just thoughts, nothing but passing mental events—we can experience a wonderful sense of freedom and ease.*

For this feature, estimate the balance of doing and being in your life (circle one):

More doing than being	Equal doing and being	More being than doing

7. Prioritizing Goal Attainment versus Sensitivity to Wider Needs

IN DOING MODE, we can become relentlessly focused on pursuing highly demanding goals and plans with a sort of tunnel vision, excluding everything else, including our own health and well-being. We may give up activities that nourish us to focus on what seems more important. Our inner resources can become depleted, leaving us feeling drained, listless, and exhausted.	*IN BEING we remain sensitive to the wider picture. Aware of the costs of a narrow focus on reaching goals, we can balance achievement with a kind and compassionate concern for our own and others' well-being. We value the quality of the moment, rather than focusing only on the distant imagined goal.*

For this feature, estimate the balance of doing and being in your life (circle one):

More doing   Equal doing   More being
than being   and being   than doing

What did you notice about the overall balance of "doing" and "being" in your life?

Chances are that, like most of us, you may have recognized that doing mode is around much of the time. The problem is that, once in doing mode, the mind can so easily slip into driven–doing: rushing from one task to another without really knowing what you are doing, often judging yourself harshly, dimly sensing there must be more to life than this. By contrast, "being mode" may seem like a far-off land, a place you rarely visit or know how to find.

Whatever you discover about how much the doing mode dominates your life, the good news is that **recognizing this** is the first step to a different way of living. Why?

Because if we can **see clearly** the different disguises in which the doing mode shows up in our daily lives, we'll see how, in feature after feature, being mode offers an alternative that will free us from the grip of the ruminative worrying mind:

- Being is a way to get out of our heads and into actually experiencing what is here in this moment—rather than endlessly thinking about it.
- Being brings acceptance to ourselves and to our experience—rather than focusing on the ways in which they fall short and need to be changed.
- Being allows us to see that thoughts don't necessarily reflect reality but are just events in the mind—in that way it strips thoughts of their power to drive our mood down further.
- As a bonus, being also allows us to be fully present with our experience of this very moment. Surprisingly, this simple shift can open a door on a whole new way to live our lives.

Where, then, does mindfulness fit into the picture?

Mindfulness

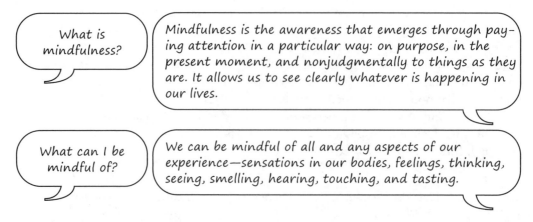

> **What is mindfulness?**
>
> Mindfulness is the awareness that emerges through paying attention in a particular way: on purpose, in the present moment, and nonjudgmentally to things as they are. It allows us to see clearly whatever is happening in our lives.

> **What can I be mindful of?**
>
> We can be mindful of all and any aspects of our experience—sensations in our bodies, feelings, thinking, seeing, smelling, hearing, touching, and tasting.

Research studies from all over the world show that the daily practice of mindfulness allows us to be fully present in our lives, improves the quality of life, and enhances our relationships.

By allowing us to be fully present, mindfulness helps us recognize and let go of habitual, automatic emotional reactions to everyday events. It provides us with a scientifically researched approach to cultivating clarity, insight, and understanding.

Mindfulness will not eliminate all of life's pain and stresses, but it can help us respond to them in a way that is kinder and more compassionate to ourselves and to those around us.

> **How do kindness and compassion fit in?**
>
> One very experienced teacher put it this way:
>
> "The quality of mindfulness is not a neutral or blank presence. True mindfulness is imbued with warmth, compassion, and interest."
>
> Kindness, warmth, and compassion are essential aspects of mindfulness if it is to transform emotional pain and suffering.

The emphasis on warmth and compassion in true mindfulness echoes the themes of approach, acceptance, and care for ourselves and others that characterize the mode of being.

Nurturing these qualities of good will counters the qualities of ill will—not wanting—that keep us stuck in emotional distress.

There are many other striking parallels between mindfulness and the being mode of mind. In fact it turns out that:

Mindfulness practice is the way to cultivate the being mode of mind.

Mindfulness Practice

Mindfulness unlocks the mind that has been imprisoned by overuse of the driven–doing mode of mind.

Mindfulness is cultivated by gently learning how to pay attention on purpose, in the present moment, and nonjudgmentally, to things as they are. This practice, also known as mindfulness *meditation,* is the core of MBCT.

Everything in the 8-week MBCT program is designed to help you become more aware of the seven signs of driven–doing and cultivate the precious human potential for mindfulness we all possess:

- We learn how to wake up from autopilot so that we don't sleep-walk through the moments of our life.
- We learn how to come close to our experience directly—rather than seeing life through thoughts narrowly focused on reaching particular goals.
- We experience a mode in which we are here, in the present moment, rather than lost in mental time travel.
- We discover firsthand how living mindfully allows us to see more clearly the little points of reactivity that can easily build into emotional turmoil. Mindfulness means we can make more conscious choices at these points—we can move from **reacting** to **responding**.
- We see how this way of being reveals a basic stance of warm kindness and compassion to ourselves and our experience.
- We learn to relate to thoughts for what they are—events in the mind—rather than as "me" or "reality."
- We nurture our capacity to nourish ourselves, rather than exhausting ourselves by striving for goals to the exclusion of all else.

In all these ways, mindfulness practice cultivates a powerful and attractive alternative to the driven–doing mode.

It pulls the plug on rumination and allows negative emotions to pass in their own time without getting us stuck in long, drawn-out misery.

Mindfulness also brings **a new way of knowing**—a direct, experiential, intuitive knowing: **knowing what we are experiencing as we are experiencing it.**

> Mindfulness means we can know our mode of mind from moment to moment. This means we can be aware when we are falling into the grip of the driven–doing mode.
>
> And, at that very moment, mindfulness itself opens the door to the healing and life-affirming qualities of being.

This new way of knowing is vital if we are to go beyond the habitual, automatic patterns of thinking, feeling, and behaving that get us trapped in ruminative thinking and cramp our wider potential to live life more fully.

Mindful awareness offers us the freedom to deliberately *choose* and shape the way we respond to life.

Mindful awareness is the heart of the MBCT program.

Chapters 2 and 3 have offered a way to understand how we get stuck in unwanted moods and how mindfulness training can get us unstuck.

In the next chapter we turn from theory to practice and look at how you might begin to get ready for that training.

Before moving on, let's reprise the key ideas covered so far:

- Emotions themselves are not the problem; the problem is the way we react to those feelings.
- Our "natural" automatic reaction to try to get rid of unpleasant feelings will often keep us stuck in the feelings. Ruminative worrying can transform passing sadness into lasting depression and fleeting fears into persistent anxiety.
- Ruminative worrying is a product of the driven–doing mode of mind, working (ineffectively) to try to get rid of feelings we don't want to have.
- We can think of driven–doing as one of a number of "mental gears" in which the mind can operate. We can free ourselves from ruminating, worrying, and getting stuck in painful emotions by learning how to "shift mental gears."

- *Being* is an alternative mental gear that provides an effective antidote to driven–doing—but few of us have been taught how to cultivate it. Cultivating the being mode of mind opens the door on a whole new way of living.
- Mindfulness training teaches us how to recognize what mental gear we are in and how to "shift gears" so that we move from driven–doing to being.
- Mindfulness training is the core of MBCT.
- MBCT is a clinically proven treatment. It also enhances our deepest capacities to live fuller, richer lives.
- MBCT works by teaching us to be more mindful, kinder, and more compassionate.

This might be a good point to take a few minutes to reflect on how MBCT might serve you:

In what ways might MBCT allow your life to unfold in line with your own deepest wishes for greater happiness and well-being?

Right now, you will probably still have unanswered questions about MBCT. Even so, is it possible to identify one reason you might wish to commit to exploring MBCT further?

Feel free to jot your thoughts down here (you may find it interesting to review this later in the light of further experience):

I intend to explore MBCT further because:

_____

_____

_____

_____

_____

_____

_____

_____

MBCT: A Brief History

Modern mindfulness-based approaches in health care began in the United States, in the late 1970s, with Jon Kabat-Zinn's development of mindfulness-based stress reduction (MBSR). His pioneering research found remarkable effects of MBSR on chronic pain and stress.

Early in the 1990s, psychologists John Teasdale and Mark Williams (from the United Kingdom) and Zindel Segal (from Canada) reasoned that mindfulness training could have powerful effects in preventing relapse in recurrent depression. On the strength of these ideas, they created the 8-week MBCT program and began to research its effectiveness. Over the past 20 years, they and others have continued this research. As a result, mindfulness has become part of mainstream evidence-based psychological treatments.

Six trials—carried out all over the world—have evaluated MBCT in depression. The results are striking. In patients with three or more previous episodes of depression, MBCT reduces the recurrence rate over 12 months by 40–50% compared with the usual treatment and has proved to be as effective as maintenance antidepressants in preventing new episodes of depression. The UK government's National Institute for Health and Clinical Excellence (NICE) has recommended it as a cost-effective treatment for preventing relapse in depression.

It is now clear that the development of MBCT was not only a highly significant advance in evidence-based therapy for recurrent depression, but also a milestone in the field of mental health, with huge potential of global significance. MBCT is a cost-effective way of reducing the risk of depression without relying on medication. It puts control back into the hands of sufferers, using practices that anyone can use, day by day, wherever they are.

Research is showing that MBCT not only prevents serious recurrent depression; it can build resilience that can help people suffering from a wide range of emotional problems: from health anxiety, social phobia, panic, and agoraphobia to bipolar disorders and chronic depression. There is also evidence that MBCT can help people deal with the psychological challenges of physical illnesses, such as cancer.

Investigations have also begun to reveal the mechanisms through which MBCT has its beneficial effects. As the theory behind MBCT predicts, increases in mindfulness in MBCT participants are one important route through which improvement occurs. Just as important, the evidence suggests, are changes in self-compassion—the way participants learn to take a gentler and friendlier attitude toward themselves—to be kinder and more compassionate and less harsh, critical, and judgmental.

One of the most exciting aspects of recent research has been the demonstration that mindfulness-based treatments can produce lasting beneficial changes in our brains. Mindfulness strengthens the brain's networks that regulate emotional reactivity, reducing the size and impact of the amygdala—the fight, flight, or freeze system; it strengthens the networks that underlie our ability to feel compassion toward ourselves and others; and it changes the pathways that normally produce habitual and unhelpful brooding whenever sad mood arises.

Getting Ready

We've looked at the ways we can get stuck in depression and other difficult emotions.

We've seen how mindfulness practice offers a way to learn how to get unstuck.

We are almost ready to begin the first week of the MBCT program.

First, let's look at some practical questions that may arise once you've decided to start:

> **Do I need to join a class to do the program in this book?**

Many people find it's helpful to attend a class if they can. It means you'll be following the program supported by the companionship and goodwill of others who also wish to embark on this journey of self-discovery. In a class you learn from others' experiences, and each member of the group helps others keep up their commitment and motivation. But if there are no classes near you, or if classes are at a time when you can't attend, it's perfectly okay to go ahead by yourself following along with this book and CD or audio downloads week by week.

> **Could my own therapist take me through the course?**

Yes. A skilled therapist or counselor, with specific experience with MBCT, can provide wonderful support and guidance as you work through the program as part of your individual therapy or counseling.

What if I'm not in therapy?

That's not a problem. You could guide yourself through the program with the help of this book, or you could ask a trusted friend or family member to be your <u>MBCT buddy</u> and do the program alongside you. Meeting up week by week with a buddy can be enormously supportive. Having the two of you working together is an invaluable way to share experiences and encourage and empower each other. And the buddy doesn't have to be facing the same difficult emotions as you—MBCT turns out to be appreciated by a wide variety of people, both with and without obvious emotional challenges.

How do I know which would be most helpful for me? A class, a therapist, a buddy, or alone?

It might be helpful to ask yourself what usually works best for you.

- Do you usually learn best by concentrating in private?
- Do you thrive and learn best with the companionship of others (with a "we're all in this together" element)?
- Do you do best on your own but with one person to have as a sounding board and friend?

Feel free to take some time to get a sense of what has worked best for you in the past and to consider following that pattern. You could always try one way now, and another way later.

Whichever way forward you choose, it's always a good idea to consider *letting friends or family know* **of your intention to complete the program, whatever it takes.** Telling people you trust of your commitment in this way can sometimes lead to support from unexpected quarters, just when it's needed most.

Nadine: "I did MBCT with a class in the next town, so at first no one at work knew—not even my best friend. I think I was afraid, deep down, of what her reaction would be. Then, at lunch one day, she mentioned she'd been getting into lots of arguments with her sister over some family thing, and it was really getting her down, and I just sort of told her how I'd been and what I'd been through and what I was doing about it—the mindfulness . . . the classes . . . all of it. She was fantastic, and we both ended up in tears."

Preparing to Get the Most Out of the Program

It's not unusual for people to find challenges coming up when they do the 8-week program.

Most people find the greatest challenge is making time.

Whether you're working with a class or on your own, the MBCT program asks you to follow along each day, 6 days out of seven, with a 40-minute mindfulness (meditation) practice—and there will be additional shorter practices to do at other times of the day as well. **In all, you should plan on finding an hour a day to practice mindfulness.**

Again and again we have been struck by the courage and commitment that participants show as they face these challenges, master them, and, almost without exception, tell us how glad they were to stay with the program all the way through to the end:

Gene: *"I found that it was really difficult at first to find the time to do the meditations. I had to get up earlier in the morning for the 8 weeks (this was hard until I decided to miss the late TV news and go to bed earlier as well). But in the end I was really glad that I gave the program the time it asked for. Not only me—everyone in the class agreed that this was the only way to gain the maximum benefit."*

Anna: *"Me too! It was really hard to find a time when the children would let me practice. I work only part-time, but the first few days were really hard. I tried getting up earlier, but my youngest seemed to have a radar system telling him I was up, and he'd wake up, get out of bed, and wander into the room and want to play . . . and he didn't seem to want to play 'meditating.' So for the first few days it felt like I was snatching time for myself. Then, I suppose it took about 10 days, I found there were times—at lunch at work, when Freddie was napping, in the evening when things were quiet—when I could do the practice we'd been given. At first I resented missing my favorite TV soap, but then I thought, 'Okay—do I want to do this program or don't I?,' and then it became less of a chore and more of an oasis."*

Like Gene and Anna, a lot of people find it difficult at first to fit in the time necessary for the program, but patience and persistence win out in the end.

This was Anna's advice:

Anna: *"Finding time isn't easy, so don't blame yourself. Try lots of things as experiments—so if it doesn't work, that's just more information rather than a reason to beat yourself up about it. Also, I am not known as Little Miss Patient, so if someone like me can persist with it (my high school teachers would be amazed!), there's a chance anyone can. Tell them it's worth it, and it's only 8 weeks."*

You might find it helpful to take a minute to think about how you will find the time the course asks you to spend in daily practice.

Here are some suggestions:

Tip: As much as possible, do the program in an 8-week stretch of your life that is free of times away on vacation, family visits, extended business trips, etc.

Tip: Do the longer meditations at the same time, and in the same place, every day.

What time of day will work best for you?

From: _____   Until: _____

Let this time be *your* time for yourself.

Tip: Tell others who need to know that you are not available to answer the door or the phone at these times.

Tip: Make a deliberate intention to protect your time for practice.

Nala: "At first I thought I was really selfish to set aside time for myself. Ken had to look after the kids, and when he wasn't around, my mom came over. But sometimes it wasn't possible, and I had to try to squeeze it in.

"One thing that a number of us noticed, though: once we had set aside the time to do it, our partners and kids really noticed the difference and liked it. It was 4 weeks in when Ken said: 'Something's changed—less "worry, worry, worry" about everything.' It's really nice. I'll never forget what he said later, a few weeks after the class had finished: 'It's lovely to have my wife back again.'"

Do protect your time for practice. Like a lioness protecting her young, please protect these times from the demands of other commitments as fiercely as you can. Remember that, for these 8 weeks, this period each day is *your* time—time for yourself to be by yourself.

If you are joining a class, enter the dates and times of the class meetings in your diary and calendar. If you are taking yourself through the program, on 1 day each week, set aside a longer period to read through the chapter that introduces the material for the upcoming week.

Being firm in carving out and protecting the time you will need for the program really pays dividends.

Remember, however . . .

If you are very depressed or life is very chaotic right now (or you are in the midst of a major change in your

life), it's probably best to wait until you are feeling a bit better, or life is a little calmer, before you begin the program.

If things are really bad right now, and you find it just too difficult to concentrate on some of the practices, it can be disheartening to struggle with new learning. It might be most skillful to allow yourself to wait a while if you can, or, if you do start, to be very gentle with yourself.

Practicalities

Finding a Place to Meditate

It's best to choose a place that feels comfortable, as quiet as practically possible, where you will not be disturbed by others or by the ringing of the phone.

Where will your place be? _____

Gathering Audio Equipment

Home practice will generally include following one or more of the guided practices recorded on the CD or using the audio downloads that accompany this book.

It might be helpful to check whether you have suitable equipment to play these guided practices.

Gathering Sitting Equipment

Sitting meditation is a central aspect of the MBCT program.

You'll see on page 75 that there are basically three options—sitting on a chair, sitting on firm cushions on the floor, or sitting on a meditation bench.

Sitting on a chair is fine, but some people find it more comfortable to use meditation cushions or a bench made for the purpose. If you think you might like to explore either of these options, now is the time to look into purchasing.

A Map of the Program

As you get ready to begin this voyage of self-discovery, you might find it helpful to have a map of the journey you will be taking; see the box on page 36.

Week by week, you will get the chance to engage with different kinds of mindfulness practice, specifically designed to address the seven core features through which the driven–doing mode of mind stands in the way of your greater peace and well-being.

Week by Week

Each week focuses on different aspects of the doing mode, so that you learn to recognize this mode and to step out of it and into the mode of being.

These are the themes you'll explore:

- Week 1—Moving from living on "automatic pilot" to living with awareness and conscious choice
- Week 2—Moving from relating to experience through thinking to directly sensing
- Week 3—Moving from dwelling in the past and future to being fully in the present moment
- Week 4—Moving from trying to avoid, escape, or get rid of unpleasant experience to approaching it with interest
- Week 5—Moving from needing things to be different to allowing them to be just as they already are
- Week 6—Moving from seeing thoughts as true and real to seeing them as mental events that may not correspond to reality
- Week 7—Moving from treating yourself harshly to taking care of yourself with kindness and compassion
- Week 8—Planning a mindful future

Each of Chapters 5–12 provides a detailed step-by-step guide.

How to Use Chapters 5–12

The chapter for each week is divided into an ORIENTATION section followed by a DAILY PRACTICE section.

We suggest using the chapters slightly differently depending on the way you are doing the course.

If you are following the course as a participant in a class:

After each weekly group session, we suggest you read through the Orientation section as a way to remind yourself of what you covered in the session.

There's no need to actually do the practices and exercises described in the Orientation section as you'll have already done them in class (although you are very welcome to do them again).

Then go on to the Daily Practice section and follow all the suggestions there.

If you are following the course as part of individual therapy or counseling:

We suggest you use each chapter as suggested by your therapist or counselor.

If you are following the course on your own or with an MBCT Buddy:

We suggest that you read the Orientation section and do all the practices and exercises described. Then go on to the Daily Practice section and follow all the suggestions there.

If you are an instructor of a group MBCT course:

This workbook will provide participants in your class with all the materials they need to complete the MBCT course.

If you would find it helpful to collect weekly summary records of participants' home practice, we recommend using the Home Practice Record Forms from *Mindfulness-Based Cognitive Therapy for Depression, Second Edition* (Segal, Williams, & Teasdale; New York: Guilford Press, 2013—download details in book).

FROM AN E-MAIL WE RECEIVED

"I feel an amazing sense of gratitude to everybody who has worked on the mindfulness for depression project.

"I reached an all-time low about 4 years ago and sought help. My counselor recommended mindfulness for me as it was evident I had experienced problems with anxiety and depression for most of my life. I read the book and listened to the CD and did the exercises and experienced rapid improvement in feelings of short-term well-being. I kept at it, and after about a year I finally got it, and day by day I am aware of my thought stream and I watch the thought buses go by without getting on them.

"This really has changed my life completely, I feel like I really understand myself a bit now, and I really have hope again, on a sustainable basis.

"I have shared this idea and process with several friends who have also benefited from it.

"I know these all sound like clichés, but I feel released from the prison/hell that was my own mind. My potential is beginning to be released at the age of 50—better late than never!

"Thank you so much, you have never met me but without wishing to be melodramatic, you have really saved my life.

"I don't know whether this will reach any of the team, or go on file as an endorsement, but I just felt the need to say thank you."

Michael

Part II

The Mindfulness-Based Cognitive Therapy (MBCT) Program

IF I HAD MY LIFE TO LIVE OVER

I'd like to make more mistakes next time.

I'd relax, I would limber up. I would be sillier than I had been on this trip. I would take fewer things seriously. I would take more chances. I would climb more mountains and swim more rivers. I would eat more ice cream and less beans. I would perhaps have more actual troubles, but I'd have fewer imaginary ones.

You see, I'm one of those people who live sensibly and sanely hour after hour, day after day. Oh, I've had my moments, and if I had to do it over again, I'd have more of them. In fact, I'd try to have nothing else. Just moments, one after another, instead of living so many years ahead of each day. I've been one of those people who never goes anywhere without a thermometer, a hot water bottle, a raincoat, and a parachute. If I had to do it again, I would travel lighter than I have.

If I had my life to live over, I would start barefoot earlier in the spring and stay that way later in the fall. I would go to more dances. I would ride more merry-go-rounds. I would pick more daisies.

Nadine Stair
85 years old
Louisville, Kentucky

5

Week 1:
Beyond Automatic Pilot

Orientation

If I had my life to live over . . . ? Depression and unhappiness—and the exhaustion and stress that come with them—all have one thing in common: they rob us of our vitality and color.

Mindfulness can help us reclaim our lives.

How do we begin?

Contrast two situations:

- Scenario 1: You're taking a walk with a young child—moving slowly, stopping often, seeing through his or her eyes the extraordinary richness of simple objects. You're seeing as if for the first time.

- Scenario 2: You're driving on a familiar route and then suddenly realize that, for miles, you have been quite unaware of your surroundings, totally lost in thought about other things. You have been "driving on automatic pilot."

These two scenarios reflect the difference between really living life as it happens and our more usual way of rushing through life—without seeing, tasting, smelling, or touching—out of touch with the world.

Just as we often "drive on automatic pilot," careful reflection reveals that we also actually "live on automatic pilot" much of the time.

The problem is that when we are out of touch in this way, the mind is not idle: it is doing what it is programmed to do—using apparent downtime to rehearse all the things we'd planned to do or daydream about what we might do.

On automatic pilot, our minds are taken over by the *doing mode*, working in the background without our knowledge, consent, or deliberate choice.

Once the doing mode has made itself at home in our minds in this way, we can easily slide into the grip of one form or another of **driven** doing—the rumination that spirals us down into another depression, the worry that traps us in anxiety, the pressing demands that make us feel ever more stressed and exhausted. Living on automatic pilot puts us at risk of getting stuck in one or other of these negative states of mind.

It also separates us from much that is positive in life, leaving us only dimly aware of the richness and fullness of life in each moment. When everything seems gray and thin, life is not much fun.

> Mindfulness offers us a way to wake up from automatic pilot.

So what can we do?

Let's begin our journey beyond automatic pilot with a new approach to a very familiar part of life—eating.

Mindfully Eating a Raisin

You will need a few raisins for this experiment in mindfulness. Settle yourself comfortably in a place where there is a good light and you will not be disturbed. Then guide yourself slowly through the practice using the instructions on audio track 2 (*Raisin Exercise*), summarized below.

**WAKING UP FROM AUTOPILOT:
AN EATING MEDITATION**

Take your time, allowing long pauses between instructions, giving at least 10 minutes to the whole meditation.

- When you are ready, take a raisin and place it on the palm of your hand . . . bring your attention to the experience of *seeing* what is on your hand. . . . Exploring the raisin with your eyes, as if you had never seen such an object before . . . bringing a wholehearted attention as you look closely and carefully . . .

- Noticing perhaps how the light hits the raisin . . . any shadows, ridges, or valleys on its surface . . . parts that are dull or glossy. . . . Allow yourself to explore it fully with your eyes. . . . Perhaps picking the raisin up with your thumb and forefinger and turning it over to explore it from all sides. . . .

- If, while you are doing this, any thoughts come to mind such as "What a strange thing I'm doing" or "What's the point of this?," then just noting them as thoughts and, as best you can, bringing your awareness back to the experience of seeing the raisin.

- And now, as you hold the raisin, bringing your full attention to the experience of touch, feeling the raisin. . . . Noticing any stickiness, or smoothness . . . if you choose, gently rolling the object between the thumb and finger, noticing parts that are soft, yielding, or more dense, sharp even. . . . Whatever you find, being aware of your experience, right now, in this moment.

- And when you're ready, bringing the raisin up to your nose and holding it there, inhaling and being aware of what you notice. . . . Noticing any perfume or aroma that might be present or, if nothing is here, noticing this as well . . . aware of any changes in your experience over time.

- And now slowly taking the raisin and preparing to place it in your mouth, aware of the changing pattern of sensations in your arm as it moves. . . . Noticing how your hand and arm know exactly where to put the raisin, perhaps closing your eyes at this point if you choose.

- Placing the raisin in your mouth, noticing if the tongue comes out to meet it . . . putting it on your tongue and allowing it to be in your mouth, but not chewing. . . . Perhaps noticing any changes inside your mouth. . . . Exploring the sensations of having the raisin on your tongue, turning the raisin over . . . exploring its surface—feeling the ridges and hollows. . . . Perhaps moving it around your mouth, to the sides . . . to the roof of the mouth.

- And when you're ready, moving the raisin between your teeth, and biting down on it . . . and, very slowly, starting to chew. . . . Noticing what is happening in your mouth . . . any taste sensations released by the chewing. . . . Taking your time. . . . Noticing any changes in your mouth and any changes in the consistency of the raisin . . . feeling the toughness of the skin . . . the softness of the flesh.

- Then, when you feel ready to swallow, seeing if you can first detect the intention to swallow as it comes up, so that even this is experienced with awareness before actually going ahead and swallowing it.

- Finally, following any sensations of swallowing, sensing the raisin moving down to your stomach and noticing the after-effects of having had the raisin in your mouth.

Now allowing your eyes to open if they have been closed and taking in the room again.

What was your experience like?

What sensations or feelings were you aware of? _____

_____

_____

_____

_____

_____

How did this differ from your normal experience of eating?

_____

_____

_____

_____

_____

Matt: "I really <u>knew</u> I was eating a raisin. The whole experience was so much more vivid than when I normally shovel a handful into my mouth at once."

Jani: "I had never even really looked at a raisin before, and this time instead of a dry wrinkly thing it looked multifaceted, like a diamond. I had to remind myself not to bite down on it at first, but exploring it with my tongue first made chewing it seem like an explosion of flavor hit my mouth."

Bringing a gentle awareness to an experience changes it. It might become richer, more interesting, or brand-new. And it shows us how unaware we are of so much that we do during a typical day.

Where did your mind go during the raisin exercise?

_____

_____

_____

_____

_____

Did you intend for your mind to go there?

If not, this is perfectly okay. It's very common to find that the mind wanders a lot. Sara almost forgot what she was doing completely:

Sara: "I don't know <u>what</u> eating the raisin was like. All I know is the fact that it looked all dried up made me think of hot sand . . . which made me think of vacations with my parents when I was a kid . . . which made me miss my mom . . . which made me think I really need to get up and call her. At that point I realized I'd swallowed the raisin and had no memory of eating it."

The mind has its own agenda. On automatic pilot, old habits of mind set the agenda and can take us places we might not choose to go.

So what does this exercise with the raisin have to do with freeing myself from getting stuck in unwanted emotions?

It's really important, actually:

1. It shows us we can change our experience just by changing the way we pay attention to it—as we will see, this gives us a whole new range of options for relating differently to unpleasant emotions.

2. It shows us that mindfulness helps us notice things that we might otherwise miss—this means we are more likely to spot the early warning signs of slipping into depression, worry, or exhaustion.

3. It shows how, on automatic pilot, thinking can take us places we might not choose to go—we can choose to come back by deliberately refocusing attention on our sense experience in this moment.

Exploring the Possibilities

Now that you've had a taste of what it's like to be newly aware during a seemingly mundane activity, you may be able to think of other daily routines you engage in on autopilot: bathing? brushing your teeth? walking from one room to another?

We'll suggest later that you write down one of these activities that you might do more mindfully, as you did with the raisin exercise, as part of daily practice this week.

The raisin exercise opens the door to mindful exploration of a whole realm of experience of which we are often unaware—our bodies. Daily practice this week brings this realm center stage in a meditation known as the Body Scan.

Daily Practice

During Week 1, practice each of these exercises **for 6 out of the next 7 days:**

1. Body Scan
2. Bringing Awareness to Routine Activities
3. Mindful Eating

1. Body Scan

Attentional Hijacking

The raisin practice shows how difficult it can be to focus on one thing for any length of time. Attention is so easily hijacked by other concerns that we don't notice how much our mind appears to have a will of its own.

Being able to focus deliberately on one thing with full attention and without distraction gives us the power to wake up from autopilot.

But most likely, like the rest of us, you haven't been taught how to train this attentional muscle.

If you're willing, you can begin this training right now. It will involve moving attention around the body. You'll learn to:

> To learn how to wake up to life, we practice three fundamental skills:
>
> - Directing attention
> - Sustaining attention
> - Shifting attention

- **direct** attention **to** the place you want it to be (engage)
- **sustain** attention so that it remains in place for the time you want it to stay (stay and explore)
- **shift** attention away when you want to (disengage).

The body scan gives you a chance to train in this way, while waking up to the actual **experience** of the body.

   Each day this week: Find a place where you can lie down comfortably for 45 minutes, without being disturbed. Follow the instructions on audio track 3 (*Body Scan*) as best you can—they're also summarized below.

BODY SCAN MEDITATION

- Lie down, making yourself comfortable, lying on your back on a mat or rug on the floor, or on your bed, in a place where you will be warm and undisturbed. Allow your eyes to close gently.

- Take a few moments to get in touch with the movement of your breath and the sensations in the body. When you are ready, bring your awareness to the physical sensations in your body, especially to the sensations of touch or pressure, where your body makes contact with the floor or bed. On each outbreath, allow yourself to let go, to sink a little deeper into the mat or bed.

- Remind yourself of the intention of this practice. Its aim is not to feel any different, relaxed or calm; this may happen or it may not. Instead, the intention of the practice is, as best you can, to bring awareness to any sensations you detect, as you focus your attention on each part of the body in turn.

- Now, bring your awareness to the physical sensations in the lower abdomen, becoming aware of the changing patterns of sensations in the abdominal wall as you breathe in and as you breathe out. Take a few moments to feel the sensations as you breathe in and as you breathe out.

- Having connected with the sensations in the abdomen, bring the focus or "spotlight" of your awareness down the left leg, into the left foot, and out to the toes of the left foot. Focus on each of the toes of the left foot in turn, bringing a gentle curiosity to investigate the quality of the sensations you find, perhaps noticing the sense of contact between the toes, a sense of tingling, warmth, or no particular sensation.

- When you are ready, on an inbreath, feel or imagine the breath entering your lungs and then passing down into the abdomen, into the left leg, the left foot, and out to the toes of the left foot. Then, on the outbreath, feel or imagine the breath coming all the way back up, out of your foot, into your leg, up through your abdomen, chest, and out through your nose. As best you can, continue this for a few breaths, breathing down into your toes and back out from your toes. It may be difficult to get the hang of this—just practice this "breathing into" as best you can, approaching it playfully.

- Now, when you are ready, on an outbreath, let go of your toes and bring awareness to the sensations on the bottom of your left foot—bringing a gentle investigative awareness to the sole of the foot, the instep, the heel (e.g., noticing the sensations where the heel makes contact with the mat or bed). Experiment with "breathing with" the sensations—being aware of the breath in the background, as, in the foreground, you explore the sensations of your lower foot.

- Now allow the awareness to expand into the rest of your foot—to the ankle, the top of the foot, and right into the bones and joints. Then, taking a slightly deeper breath, directing it down into the whole of your left foot, and, as the breath lets go on the outbreath, let go of the left foot completely, allowing the focus of awareness to move into your lower left leg—the calf, shin, knee, and so on, in turn.

- Continue to bring awareness, and a gentle curiosity, to the physical sensations in each part of the rest of your body in turn—to the upper left leg, the right toes, right foot, right leg, pelvic area, back, abdomen, chest, fingers, hands, arms, shoulders, neck, head, and face. In each area, as best you can, bring the same detailed level of awareness and gentle curiosity to the bodily sensations present. As you leave each major area, "breathe in" to it on the inbreath and let go of that region on the outbreath.

- When you become aware of tension or of other intense sensations in a particular part of the body, you can "breathe in" to them—using the inbreath gently to bring awareness right into the sensations, and, as best you can, have a sense of their letting go, or releasing, on the outbreath.

- The mind will inevitably wander away from the breath and the body from time to time. That is entirely normal. It is what minds do. When you notice it, gently acknowledge it, noticing where the mind has gone off to, and then gently return your attention to the part of the body you intended to focus on.

- After you have "scanned" the whole body in this way, spend a few minutes being aware of a sense of the body as a whole and of the breath flowing freely in and out of the body.

- If you find yourself falling asleep, you might find it helpful to prop your head up with a pillow, open your eyes, or do the practice sitting up rather than lying down. Feel free to experiment with doing the practice at a different time of day.

Each day, **write a few notes** in the spaces provided about what you were most aware of during the body scan. What were you **thinking**? What **sensations in your body** did you notice? What **emotions or feelings** did you experience?

Day 1:

Thoughts

_____

_____

Sensations

_____

_____

Feelings

_____

_____

I kept thinking, Am I doing this right? Am I trying hard enough? Why can't I relax? Why isn't anything happening?

That's actually quite a common experience. All these thoughts are just different forms of judging—driven-doing mind wheeling in to take over the action. As best you can, just say "judging" gently to yourself and bring the attention back to the region of the body that the instructions are focusing on in that moment.

There is no "right" way for the body scan to be.
Our experience is our experience, however that may be.

Day 2:

Thoughts

_____

_____

Sensations

_____

_____

Feelings

_____

_____

It didn't do anything for me. I just kept falling _asleep_.

It's easy for that to happen. See if it's possible to just keep doing the body scan, day after day, even if it seems that to begin with you are spending more time asleep than awake. Often, over time, the sleepiness gets less. If it persists, you might try doing the body scan with your eyes open or prop your head up with a pillow or do the practice sitting up. If you have been practicing in the evenings, you might experiment with doing it earlier in the day.

Day 3:

Thoughts

_____

_____

Sensations

_____

_____

Feelings

_____

_____

It was amazing—I felt so _relaxed_, it was as if parts of my body were fading away. It was wonderful, as if I weighed nothing at all.

How lovely! When this happens, it can give us confidence that we already have the possibilities for peace and calm deep within us. But it's helpful to be careful about expecting or wishing for this to happen next time—it may or it may not. Although relaxation is not the real point of the body scan, it's fine to enjoy it if it happens.

Perhaps surprisingly, the aim of the body scan
isn't to strive for relaxation, or any other special state.
It doesn't matter what sensations you become aware of—
the important thing is that, as best you can, you tune in
to the *direct sense* of the body rather than getting entangled
in *thinking about* it.

Day 4:

Thoughts

_____

_____

Sensations

_____

_____

Feelings

_____

_____

I couldn't focus. I kept thinking, "How can I meditate with all this going on?"—with the kids running around and the phone ringing, and people banging on the door. I'd get so <u>frustrated</u> that I wasn't getting anywhere with all the time I'm spending on this.

When you experience frustration, irritation, or boredom, see if it's possible to just acknowledge these emotions for what they are—passing states of mind—perhaps saying to yourself "here's frustration," "here's boredom," etc.— and then, rather than trying to get rid of these emotions, simply coming back to the practice, bringing your attention to the instructions and wherever they are inviting you to focus your awareness.

Day 5:

Thoughts

_____

_____

Sensations

_____

_____

Feelings

_____

_____

I tried to relax, but I kept noticing <u>tension and aches</u>. If it doesn't feel pleasant, I can't be doing it right, can I? It's really <u>uncomfortable</u>.

With mindfulness, we can become very aware of what's happening in our bodies. If you experience discomfort, as best you can, let go of judging whether or not you are doing the practice "right" and simply focus your attention where the instructions suggest. Then, when the instructions get to the area that is tense or uncomfortable, explore those physical sensations as gently as you can. And when the instructions move on, release the attention and refocus it in the new region. . . . You may find it helpful to remember that you don't need to feel good <u>now</u> for this training to be nourishing your capacity for stillness and clarity—those effects may well show up at other times.

Day 6:

Thoughts

_____

_____

Sensations

_____

_____

Feelings

_____

_____

> I found myself in floods of tears, and I just couldn't understand why.

> When we tune in to the sensations in the body, we may reconnect with emotions that, at some time, the mind chose not to fully experience. Although this can be startling, the willingness to allow such feelings to be present can be profoundly healing. To the extent you can, see if it's possible to continue to follow the instructions and focus on the body sensations of the moment. That way, you "steady" yourself in the face of <u>strong emotion</u>.

If you find yourself *repeatedly* reconnecting with
overwhelming emotions from a past traumatic experience,
or you find memories of extremely distressing events
coming back, it is wise to seek further professional help—
from your MBCT instructor (if you have one)
or from an experienced counselor or therapist.

At the end of the week you might like to reflect on your own experience of the following common reactions to the practice. Circle any that you noticed and jot down any specific experiences that stuck in your mind:

Judging

_____

_____

Sleepiness

_____

_____

Calm/Relaxation

_____

_____

Physical Discomfort

_____

_____

Frustration/Boredom

_____

_____

Emotional Upset

_____

_____

Other (specify)

_____

_____

_____

_____

_____

_____

_____

_____

_____

_____

LOOKING BACK:
A PARTICIPANT IN MBCT LOOKS BACK ON THE BODY SCAN

For the first 10 days it was like a burden. I kept wandering off, and then I would worry about whether I was doing it right. For example, I kept having flights of fantasy. My mind was all over the place. I tried too hard to stop it, I think.

Another problem at the start was him saying "Just accept things as they are now." I thought that was totally unreasonable. I thought to myself, I can't do that.

Eventually, I just put the CD on and expected to go off into a realm of thoughts. I didn't worry if concerns came in. Gradually the 40 minutes passed without me losing him, and from then on, the next time was more effective.

After ten days I relaxed more. I stopped worrying about whether I was thinking about anything else. When I stopped worrying about it, I actually stopped the flights of fantasy. If I did think of something else, I picked up the CD again when I stopped thinking. Gradually the flights of fantasy reduced. I was happy to listen to him, and then I started to get some value from it.

Soon I had developed it so that I could actually feel the breath going down to the base of my foot. Sometimes I didn't feel anything, but then I thought, If there's no feeling, I can be satisfied with the fact there is no feeling.

It's not something you can do half a dozen times. It's got to be a daily thing. It becomes more real the more that you try it. I began to look forward to it.

If people have got to structure the time for the 45 minutes for their practice, it may be easier to structure other things in their life as well. The practice in itself would provide an impetus.

2. Bringing Awareness to Routine Activities

Practicing mindfulness in everyday life is a central aspect of the MBCT program. There are two ways to begin to do that this week. The first is bringing mindful awareness to a routine activity.

It's important to practice being mindful in our everyday lives because that's where we need it.

Choose *one routine activity* you do every day and resolve that this week you will bring to it, as best you can, a fresh quality of deliberate and gentle moment-to-moment awareness, just as you did with the raisin. It's best to stay with the same activity each day for the whole week.

You could use one of the activities you thought of earlier or something else, such as one of these possibilities:

waking up in the morning	taking out the garbage
drying your body	driving the car
getting dressed	leaving the house
making coffee	entering the house
washing the dishes	going upstairs
loading the dishwasher	going downstairs

> I'm not sure what deliberate awareness feels like. What should I pay attention to?

> It's really good to get this clear. Let's say you choose showering, for example. Then you would pay wholehearted attention to the sensations on your skin as the water makes contact, the warmth of the water, the smell of the shampoo or soap, the sound of the water, and the shifting sensations in the muscles of the arms as you move them to wash your body.

> Another example—if you choose waking, before you get out of bed, see if it's possible to feel the sensations of touch and pressure where your body contacts the mattress and bedclothes, to pay gentle attention to the movements of the breath for five inbreaths and five outbreaths, to open your awareness to the sounds of the morning, to feel the air on your face, and to notice what you see around you.

See if it is possible to gently **wake up** to your experience
of life and know what you are doing directly,
as you are doing it.

Everyday Activity for Week 1: _____

To keep track of this practice, every day, make a ✓ whenever you remember to be mindful of the activity:

Day 1: _____   Day 2: _____   Day 3: _____

Day 4: _____   Day 5: _____   Day 6: _____

In itself, mindfulness is not difficult—the challenge in everyday life for all of us is **remembering** to be mindful. Is there any pattern in the times when you remember and the times you forget?

It's **easier** to remember when:

_____

_____

It's **more difficult** to remember when:

_____

_____

At the end of the week: Reflect a moment on any differences you noticed between the way you experienced your chosen activity this week and your normal experience:

_____

_____

_____

_____

_____

Jani: *"Once I started being mindful of ordinary moments during my day I found myself noticing all sorts of little things—a bird flying across the sky, the smell as I cooked dinner, the crackling sound as I strode through fallen leaves. When I was really aware of these things, I didn't brood about worries."*

Georgios: *"Paying more attention to the whole process of waking up in the morning and getting out of bed seemed to make the mild depressed feeling that I always wake up with lift more quickly."*

Bringing awareness to the activities of daily living makes it easier to recognize when we are in doing mode or on automatic pilot.

It also provides us with a way to immediately switch modes of mind and deliberately enter and dwell in the mode of being, where it's harder for depression or other troubling emotions to take hold.

3. Mindful Eating

The second exercise in bringing mindfulness into daily life this week is mindful awareness of eating.

This exercise invites you to **become aware** of times when you find that you are noticing the tastes, sights, smells, or body sensations as you are eating—just like you did when you were mindfully eating the raisin.

See if it's also possible to eat at least one meal, or part of a meal, mindfully—giving it the same care and attention as when you ate the raisin.

Make a ✓ every time you notice you are eating mindfully (it's fine to enter more than one ✓ if you are mindful of more than one meal or snack per day).

Day 1: _____   Day 2: _____   Day 3: _____

Day 4: _____   Day 5: _____   Day 6: _____

At the end of the week, you might like to **reflect** on any changes in your eating. Jot down your thoughts here:

_____

_____

_____

_____

_____

Congratulations!

You have reached the end of Week 1 of the MBCT program.

It might be helpful and interesting at this point to look back over your notes as a reminder of the experience of the week as a whole—how you responded to each practice and how your reactions and responses may have been different from one day to the next.

Your reactions in Week 2 may be similar to those from Week 1, or they may be very different. There's only one way to find out. Are you ready?

You Reading This, Be Ready

Starting here, what do you want to remember?
How sunlight creeps along a shining floor?
What scent of old wood hovers, what softened
sound from outside fills the air?

Will you ever bring a better gift for the world
than the breathing respect that you carry
wherever you go right now? Are you waiting
for time to show you some better thoughts?

When you turn around, starting here, lift this
new glimpse that you found; carry into evening
all that you want from this day. This interval you spent
reading or hearing this, keep it for life—

What can anyone give you greater than now,
starting here, right in this room, when you turn around?

WILLIAM STAFFORD

6

Week 2:
Another Way of Knowing

Orientation

Valerie: *"It's so difficult to stay focused in the body scan! I lie down, determined that, this time, I'm going to follow the instructions exactly. And yet, a minute into the practice, I find I'm thinking about my body, wondering why I feel so many aches I haven't noticed before, wondering what it all might mean. Eventually I realize I've lost contact with my body <u>again</u>, and I turn on myself: 'This is so simple, why can't I just do it right? Others can do this. What's wrong with me?' It's just like when I tried to learn Spanish—the stuff just wouldn't go in. I really felt stupid on that trip to Mexico. . . .*

"I end up spending the rest of the session thinking about other times I've messed up and what it all means about the kind of person I really am.

"By the end of the session I end up feeling worse than when I started."

On autopilot, it is as if we are away somewhere. But where do we go? Most often, we are lost in thinking of one form or another—planning, remembering, or daydreaming.

Thinking becomes a problem when it takes over—when we are no longer just thinking, but **lost** in thought. We've passed a tipping point: no longer living in the world, we are living in our heads.

So what do we do? We can't stop thinking simply by using willpower. And we still need to know what's going on, right now, in our lives. Is there a different way, other than thinking, for us to know, and relate to, our experience?

Try an experiment; you'll find the instructions for it below, or, if you prefer, on audio track 14 (*Two Ways of Knowing*). It will take just a few minutes.

> The thinking of the doing mind underlies the rumination of depression, the worry of anxiety, and the restless striving of the stressed-out state.

TWO WAYS OF KNOWING

Settle yourself into a comfortable position on an upright chair. Close your eyes.

1. Thinking *About*

Take a minute or two to **think about** your feet without looking at them. What thoughts arise when you bring your feet to mind? There might be thoughts of liking or disliking, of wanting them to be different . . . thoughts of where they've taken you or problems they've caused you . . . thoughts of—what?

There's no need to control your thinking in any way—just let the thinking unfold naturally. Take your time; give yourself a minute or two to think about your feet.

2. Tuning In Directly

Next, bring your attention right **into** your feet without looking at them—allow **awareness** to sink into and fill your feet from inside to outside . . . from the bones right out to the skin itself . . . sensing the bones within the feet . . . feeling the sensations of touch on the skin. . . . the sensations in the soles of the feet . . . the sense of touch, pressure, and contact where the feet touch the floor . . . exploring the boundary between the feet and the floor.

Now clench your toes a little, drawing them in as close as you can, paying attention to the physical sensations in the toes, soles, and body of each foot . . . directly sensing the pressures in the toes . . . feeling the tightness in the muscles, the flux and flow of bodily sensations throughout the feet, ankles, and legs.

And now, just ease the grip of the toes, keeping the awareness in your feet, noticing the changes in the sensations in the feet and toes as they relax.

Finally, before you change position, take a few moments to get a sense of your body as a whole, sitting here.

What did you notice while you were **thinking about** your feet? Jot down a few notes here:

_____

_____

_____

_____

_____

Valerie: "Thinking about my feet reminded me how very tired I have been feeling lately—how at times it feels like such an effort just to put one foot in front of the other. It brought back memories: of times I've been dead on my feet from working too hard, of my dad with his gnarled and deformed feet when he got old. I began to wonder what the future holds for me--weariness, old age, illness. It made me quite sad."

Thinking and memory, central to the DOING mode's way of knowing, can take us a long way from the immediacy of present experience.

What did you notice when you tuned in **directly** to the sensations in your feet?

_____

_____

_____

_____

Valerie: "At first I noticed a sense of warmth throughout my feet. Then there was a sense of tingling in the toes—it came and went as I focused attention on the sensations. When I clenched my toes, all the sensations in my feet became much stronger and easier to tune in to; they were intense but not unpleasant. With my right foot particularly, I was really interested in the way the sensations from my foot did not feel foot-shaped—I'd never noticed that before. At the end, I was aware my mind had been quite focused, not wandering as it did when I thought about my feet."

Directly sensing the body weakens the chatter of the mind. The direct knowing of the BEING mode means we can stay closer to immediate, bare experience and are less likely to be carried away by thought.

What, for you, was the most striking difference between the two ways of knowing—thinking *about* your feet versus placing your attention *inside* the sensations of your feet?

_____

_____

_____

_____

_____

In doing mode we **know about** our experience only indirectly, through thought. In this mode we can easily get lost in rumination and worry.

Through mindfulness we discover another kind of knowing—a quieter, wiser voice that is usually drowned out by the louder shouts of the thinking mind.

In this **direct** relating to experience we are simply aware of our experience in the moment—**the knowing is in the awareness itself**.

When we mindfully encounter something unpleasant, rather than having ideas about it, we relate to it **as experience**—sensing it, feeling it. There is a beautiful simplicity in this knowing. It allows us to connect, immediately, with a greater freedom and ease.

> When we find we are lost in thinking, refocusing attention to become directly aware of sensations in our bodies provides a way to release ourselves from the world of thought.

This week, you are invited to practice recognizing when you become lost in thought and then reconnecting with direct, mindful knowing of the body.

Every time you notice the mind has wandered offers an opportunity to practice shifting from living in your head to directly sensing your body.

To understand the liberating power of that shift from one way of knowing to another, let's look more closely at why knowing-by-thinking can be such a problem.

The Hidden Power of Thinking: Thoughts and Feelings

THE "WALKING DOWN THE STREET" EXERCISE

Settle into a comfortable position. When you are ready, read through the scenario described below. Take a minute or two to imagine the scene as vividly as you can. You may find it helpful to close your eyes. Take all the time you need—see if it is possible to engage fully with the imagined scene.

> You are walking along a familiar street . . . You see someone you know on the other side of the street . . . You smile and wave . . . The person makes no response . . . just doesn't seem to notice you . . . walks past without any sign of recognizing your existence.
>
> Imagine that scene now.

What thoughts and feelings went through your mind?

_____

_____

_____

_____

_____

How do I distinguish my thoughts from my feelings?

They're both aspects of inner experience, so the difference can be difficult to put into words. But thoughts are what we often experience as words and sentences going through the mind, or as pictures or images that are fairly easy to describe with words, whereas feelings are more like sensations or shifts in emotional state that are experienced directly. The table below, which shows some typical responses to this exercise, may make things clearer.

	Thoughts	Feelings
Carol	*"He didn't even acknowledge me. What did I do to upset him?"*	*Worried*
Jake	*"I wonder how that happened."*	*Curious*
Sharon	*"She doesn't like me. Nobody really likes me."*	*Depressed*
Betsy	*"You must have seen me. Fine, if that's how you feel. Do what you want."*	*Angry*
Lena	*"She was probably preoccupied with something. I hope she's okay."*	*Concerned*

The table shows the responses of a number of different people to exactly the same exercise that you've just done. Does anything strike you about them? You might like to go back and have another look at them—they reveal some crucially important truths about the way our minds and hearts work. Jot down anything that strikes you about them here.

_____

_____

_____

You may have noticed that the thoughts in the table varied from person to person and that different thoughts went with different feelings. Exactly the same situation can call forth a wide range of thoughts and interpretations, and **it is these, rather than the situation itself**, that shape the way we feel: if we think someone is ignoring us because we have done something wrong, we feel upset; if we think someone is deliberately ignoring us, we feel angry; if we think the person is preoccupied with his own worries, we feel concern; and so on. But, crucially, **we are often unaware of our interpretations** of situations. Mindfulness can help us become more aware and give us the freedom to respond differently.

Our emotional reactions reflect the interpretations we give to situations rather than the situations themselves.

It might also have struck you that even though they all heard the same scene being described, it was as if each person actually experienced a different situation in his or her mind's eye.

Our interpretations of events reflect what we bring to them just as much as the reality of the events themselves.

The thoughts are our interpretations, the conclusions we draw, often based on preconceived notions and prior experiences, and so they are shaped by a lot of different influences. The fact that people had such different interpretations means these thoughts cannot all be accurate reflections of the same reality—they cannot all be right. There will often be no simple one-to-one relationship between how things actually are and what we think.

Thoughts are not facts—they are mental events.

I've noticed I interpret the same experience differently at different times. Why is that?

Moods powerfully bias the way we see things. In a depressed mood we interpret events negatively—we think someone is deliberately ignoring us rather than that she might be preoccupied with troubles of her own. These negative interpretations—"She doesn't like me; what have I done wrong?"—make us feel more depressed. This makes us more likely to continue to see things negatively, and down we spiral.

Similarly, if we are feeling tense and anxious, our minds are tuned to see things that can go wrong, or threaten us, or that <u>have</u> to be done. All these just make us more tense, anxious, and stressed—and on and on it goes.

Our moods affect how we interpret events in ways
that keep the moods going.

The spirals in which thoughts and moods feed off each other are what lock us into emotional distress and depression—*it is our thinking that gets us stuck.*

We can step out of the thinking patterns that keep us gripped in painful emotions by switching our way of knowing—from being lost in our heads to knowing and sensing our bodies directly, mindfully. That's the practice for this week.

Daily Practice

During Week 2, practice each of these exercises **for 6 out of the next 7 days**:

1. Body Scan
2. Mindfulness of Breathing (Brief)
3. Bringing Awareness to Routine Activities
4. Pleasant Experiences Calendar

1. Body Scan

> *Didn't I do this last week? Why am I doing it again?*

> *The practice is the same, but the experience will be different every day. As much as possible, approach each body scan with a fresh, open mind, acknowledging that you've never done THIS body scan before, so who knows what each new moment may have to offer?*
>
> *We continue this practice because the doing mode is such an old and well-established habit that it takes a lot of patience and persistence both to train the mind to be where you want it to be and to cultivate the direct knowing of the being mode.*

The Body Scan

- gives us a great way of training our attentional muscle: moving through the *"engage–remain–disengage"* cycle many times
- helps us get back in touch with our bodies and out of our heads

---

Each day this week Find a place where you can lie down comfortably and follow the instructions on pages 47–48 or on audio track 3 (*Body Scan*).

Immediately after each practice, **jot down a few notes** on your experience in the spaces provided.

What thinking patterns did you experience as the doing mode took over your mind? Planning and rehearsing? Blame and judgment? Wanting to hurry up? Reminders of unfinished business? Going back over things from the past?

What was your response? Were you able to ease back into being mode, or did you stay stuck in doing? What else did you notice?

Day 1:

What forms of doing did you notice (e.g., planning, hurrying up, judging, unfinished business, going over the past?): _____

_____

_____

Response: _____

_____

_____

I also noticed: _____

_____

_____

> I kept thinking, This is boring. Nothing's happening.

> You might like to see if it's possible to be aware of this simply as a thinking pattern—"judging"—rather than getting drawn into it and lost inside it. You can then gently shift from thinking about your experience to directly sensing it by bringing an interested awareness to the sensations in your body.

Each time we notice we have been lost in thinking offers a precious opportunity to practice the move from doing to being—that is the way to freedom.

Day 2:

Doing (e.g., planning, hurrying up, judging, unfinished business, going over the past?): _____

_____

_____

Response: _____

_____

_____

I also noticed: _____

_____

_____

I stayed awake for the whole session for the first time!

Great! Our experience is always changing—if you look carefully, you will see that your experience of this practice (and all other practices) is never the same from one day to the next. The body scan has powerful effects, but they build slowly over time. Keep going!

Day 3:

Doing (e.g., planning, hurrying up, judging, unfinished business, going over the past?): _____

_____

_____

Response: _____

_____

_____

I also noticed: _____

_____

_____

I'm getting more relaxed about the whole thing. If I notice I'm lost in thought, I don't give myself such a hard time—somehow, that seems to weaken the pull of the thoughts.

That's a nice observation. When we don't take our thoughts so seriously, they have less "charge" and don't demand our attention so greedily. We may even find we can just let them be there, gently, in the background, while we focus back to the sensations in the body.

It can be really helpful to remember that kindness is the foundation for all skillful practice.

Day 4:

Doing (e.g., planning, hurrying up, judging, unfinished business, going over the past?): _____

_____

_____

Response: _____

_____

_____

I also noticed: _____

_____

_____

Sometimes I wonder whether all this effort is worthwhile—whether this course is what I need, whether I can do it. Not much seems to have happened yet.

This is <u>doubting mind</u>—a very common pattern of thinking at this stage in the program—this kind of thinking reflects a state of mind, not a true view of how things really are. At the end of the course, when we ask participants who have had doubts like this what advice we should give to others with similar doubts, they always say "Just tell them to keep going, regardless—they will not regret it."

Day 5:

Doing (e.g., planning, hurrying up, judging, unfinished business, going over the past?): _____

_____

_____

Response: _____

_____

_____

I also noticed: _____

_____

_____

> I find I'm beginning to look forward to my body scan sessions. It feels like a time for me, when I can take a break from my mind and rest in my body for a while.

> Absolutely! The driven–doing mind can drive us so hard—"do this," "do that," "don't forget to," "be sure to do this properly." Mindfulness of our bodies offers a refuge and haven that is always there for us with a simple shift of attention.

Day 6:

Doing (e.g., planning, hurrying up, judging, unfinished business, going over the past?): _____

_____

_____

Response: _____

_____

_____

I also noticed: _____

_____

_____

> I'm feeling bad because I'm not doing the practice every day. Somehow I never get around to it, and by the time I think of it, there's no time.

> Once the judging self-critical mind gets on the case, it's easy to get trapped in a vicious cycle:
> <u>Self-blame</u> → negative associations with practice → <u>avoid</u> practice → <u>more self-blame</u> → less practice . . .
> The good news is that, in any moment, we can always wipe the slate clean, let go of what has happened, and begin again.

Whatever has happened in the past, we can always begin again, right now, by actually *doing* the practice, rather than *dwelling* on our previous failures to practice.

ADAM

Adam had been feeling down for a week or two. Each day, as he awoke, he noticed the sense of heaviness and achiness in his body. He felt drained of energy, unrefreshed by his night's sleep, sometimes even more tired than when he went to bed. Usually this sense of weariness triggered a familiar chorus of thoughts: "How am I going to get anything done feeling like this?" "Another wasted day." "I can't go on like this." "What's going to happen to me?"

And with these thoughts came a sense of frustration and defeat. These just added to the sense of burden and heaviness in Adam's body. Eventually, somehow, he would struggle out of bed and make a reluctant start to his day, worrying about where it was all going to lead.

After 10 days' practice of the body scan, Adam began to recognize the difference between the "knowing by thinking" of the doing mode and the direct "knowing by awareness" of the being mode.

And then, remembering something that had been said in his MBCT class, it occurred to Adam to try the same practice when he woke in the morning: What would happen if he directly sensed the heaviness and achiness in his body rather than spiraled off into thinking about them?

It made a difference—not a miracle cure—but Adam found it just a little easier to stay present in the moment with his experience, uncomfortable as it was. And, interestingly, being willing to be there for his experience, knowing it directly in that way, meant that his energy increased, rather than dwindled further away. He didn't exactly bound joyfully out of bed, but he found he didn't lie there quite as long as usual, and he approached his day a little lighter in spirits.

At the end of Week 2, you might like to take a few moments to reflect on your experience of the body scan as a whole over the last two weeks.

The body scan will not be included in daily practice for the next few weeks, so this is an opportunity to close the book on this practice for now.

Reflecting on your experience, what is ONE thing you have learned from the body scan practice?

_____

_____

_____

_____

2. Mindfulness of Breathing (Brief)

Mindfulness of breathing—a *sitting meditation*—is a core practice in the MBCT program. It takes center stage from next week onward.

This week we introduce this practice with a brief daily exercise.

Each day, at a different time from the body scan, guide yourself through a 10-minute mindfulness of the breath practice, using the instructions on audio track 4 (*10-Minute Sitting Meditation*), summarized below. Feel free to copy the helpful hints on page 75 or download them from *www.guilford.com/teasdale-materials* to have them at hand.

10-MINUTE MINDFULNESS OF BREATHING (SITTING) MEDITATION

1. Settle into a comfortable sitting position, allowing your back to adopt an erect, dignified, and comfortable posture—not stiff but a posture that embodies your intention to be present and awake. If sitting on a chair, place your feet flat on the floor, with your legs uncrossed. Gently close your eyes.

2. Bring your awareness to the level of *physical sensations* by focusing your attention on the *sensations* of touch and pressure in your body where it makes contact with the floor and whatever you are sitting on. Spend a minute or two exploring these sensations, just as in the body scan.

3. Now bring your awareness to the *changing patterns of physical sensations* in your lower abdomen (in the area around the navel) as the breath moves in and out of your body. (When you first try this practice, it may be helpful to place your hand on your lower abdomen and become aware of the *changing pattern of sensations* where your hand makes contact with your abdomen. Having tuned in to the *physical sensations* in this area in this way, you can remove your hand and continue to focus on the *sensations* in the abdominal wall.)

4. Focus your awareness on the *sensations* of slight stretching as the abdominal wall rises with each inbreath and of gentle deflation as it falls with each outbreath. As best you can, follow with your awareness the *changing physical sensations* in the lower abdomen all the way through as the breath enters your body on the inbreath and all the way through as the breath leaves your body on the outbreath, perhaps noticing the slight pauses between one inbreath and the following outbreath and between one outbreath and the following inbreath.

5. There is no need to try to control your breathing in any way—simply let the breath breathe itself. As best you can, also bring this attitude of allowing to the rest of your experience. There is nothing to be fixed, no particular state to be achieved. As best you can, simply allow your experience to be your experience, without needing it to be other than it is.

6. Sooner or later (usually sooner), your mind will wander away from the focus on the breath in the lower abdomen to thinking, planning, daydreaming, drifting along—whatever. This is perfectly okay—it's simply what minds do. It is not a mistake or a failure. When you notice that your awareness is no longer on the breath, gently congratulate yourself—you have come back and are once more aware of your experience! You may want to acknowledge briefly where your mind has been ("Ah, here's thinking"). Then gently escort your awareness back to a focus on the changing pattern of physical sensations in the lower abdomen, renewing the intention to pay attention to the ongoing inbreath or outbreath, whichever you find.

7. No matter how often you notice that your mind has wandered (and this will quite likely happen over and over again), as best you can, congratulate yourself each time on reconnecting with your experience in the moment, gently escorting your attention back to the breath, and simply resume awareness of the changing pattern of physical sensations that come with each inbreath and outbreath.

8. As best you can, bring a quality of kindliness to your awareness, perhaps seeing the repeated wanderings of the mind as opportunities to bring patience and gentle curiosity to your experience.

9. Continue with the practice for 10 minutes, or longer if you wish, perhaps reminding yourself from time to time that the intention is simply to be aware of your experience in each moment, as best you can. Using the breath as an anchor, gently reconnect with the here and now each time you notice that your mind has wandered and is no longer down in the abdomen, following your breath.

There's no need, this week, to make notes on your experience with this practice—we'll be focusing on it in detail in Week 3.

Just make a ✓ each day to show yourself you've done the practice:

Day 1: _____   Day 2: _____   Day 3: _____

Day 4: _____   Day 5: _____   Day 6: _____

Sitting Meditation: Helpful Hints

- It's worth taking some time to find a sitting position that works for you. The idea is to find a comfortable, stable sitting position, with your back erect but not stiff.

- It's fine to use a chair—there's nothing special about sitting on the floor, although some people find it more comfortable. If you use a chair, choose one that has a straight back and allows your feet to be flat on the floor with your legs uncrossed. It is best, if you can, to sit well away from the back of the chair so that your spine is self-supporting.

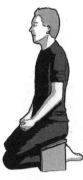

- If you sit on a soft surface on the floor, use a firm, thick cushion, or a meditation bench or stool, that raises your bottom three to six inches off the floor and allows your knees to touch the floor. You have the choice of three different ways to sit:

  Option 1: on a cushion, drawing one heel in close to your body and folding your other leg in front of it

  Option 2: kneeling with a cushion between your feet

  Option 3: sitting on a meditation bench or stool

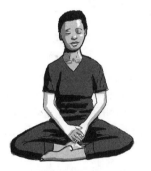
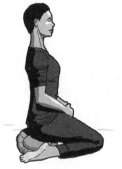
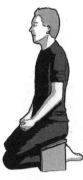

Option 1 **Option 2** **Option 3**

Experiment with the height of the cushions or bench until you feel comfortable and firmly supported.

*Whatever you sit on, arrange things so that your knees
are lower than your hips.*

When you sit with your knees lower than your hips, your lower back will have a gentle inward curve and your spine will be self-supporting. Rest your hands in your lap or on your thighs.

Many people find a bench the ideal way to get the right posture—you can experiment with adding cushions or a folded blanket to get the height just right for you.

3. Bringing Awareness to Routine Activities

Remind yourself of the daily activity to which you chose to bring mindfulness last week by writing it here:

_____ (Activity 1)

Now choose a new and different routine activity that you can also include in the scope of this practice of daily mindfulness:

_____ (Activity 2)

By making a deliberate intention to bring mindfulness to **both** these activities this week you can reinforce and extend your commitment to be mindful in everyday life.

Every day, make a ✓ whenever you remember to be mindful of Activity 1 **or** Activity 2:

Day 1: _____   Day 2: _____   Day 3: _____

Day 4: _____   Day 5: _____   Day 6: _____

At the end of the week, take a few moments to reflect on your experience of this practice as a whole. It won't be part of assigned home practice from now on, but many people find they like to extend this practice on their own. Can you think of **one positive effect** that might make you want to continue deliberately cultivating the intention to be mindfully present with the daily activities of your life?:

_____

_____

_____

_____

_____

_____

_____

Roy: *"Yesterday evening my two young daughters were playfully heaping as many sofa cushions on my head as they could while I sat desperately trying to read a paper for work. I managed to muster a smile at their persistence, but in my failure to concentrate on the paper, I found my mind constantly jumping from one thing to the next. This is usually my trigger to have a mindful moment, so I refocused and gave myself fully to being with my two girls. The next five minutes were the most rewarding and most meaningful five minutes of being a parent that I can recall for several weeks."*

4. Pleasant Experiences Calendar

Each day, aim to be aware of one pleasant experience **as it is happening**.

The experience can be quite ordinary, something as simple as hearing a bird sing or noticing the smile on the face of a child; the important thing is that it has a pleasant feel to it.

There are two parts to this practice:

1. Consciously choosing **what** you pay attention to—by looking out for pleasant experiences
2. Consciously choosing **how** you pay attention, by focusing on the separate aspects of each pleasant experience—the pleasant feeling itself and any other feelings around, any thoughts going through your mind, and the sensations in your body

Use the following questions to focus your awareness on the details of the experience as it is happening. You can write it down later.

What was the experience?	What sensations did you feel in your body, in detail?	What moods or feelings did you notice?	What thoughts went through your mind?	What thoughts are in your mind now as you write this down?
Example: Heading home at the end of my shift— stopping, hearing a bird sing	Lightness across the face, aware of shoulders dropping, uplift of corners of mouth	Relief, pleasure	"That's good," "How lovely [the bird is]," "It's so nice to be outside."	"It was such a small thing, but I'm glad I noticed it."

Make your descriptions fairly detailed—for example, write down your thoughts word for word if that's how you experience them or describe any images in your mind's eye; note exactly where any sensations were felt in the body and what they were. Use the act of recording itself as an opportunity to become aware of any thoughts going through your mind as you write.

Day 1 *What was the experience?*	*What sensations did you feel in your body, in detail?*	*What moods or feelings did you notice?*	*What thoughts went through your mind?*	*What thoughts are in your mind now as you write this down?*

Knowing-by-thinking means we see experiences as blobs—things that are either good or bad in themselves and that we have to hang on to or get rid of to be happy. This is the driven–doing mode of mind.

Focusing attention on the separate aspects of experience—body sensations, feelings, thoughts—allows us to "de-blob," to relate to experience as constantly shifting patterns that we can simply know directly in the moment. When we relate to experience in this way, we pull the plug on the driven-doing mode of mind.

Day 2 *Experience?*	*Sensations, in detail?*	*Moods or feelings?*	*Thoughts then?*	*Thoughts now?*

Many of us end up tuning out unpleasant feelings as a way of self-protection. In the long run, this simply doesn't work. It also means we numb out more generally from **all** feelings—unpleasant **and** pleasant. In this way, we cut ourselves off from much of the potential richness of life and from our mind and heart's deep potential for healing. Paying attention directly to the simple sense of whether an experience is pleasant or not can reconnect us with the wider world of feeling and open us more fully to the wonder of being alive.

Day 3 *Experience?*	*Sensations, in detail?*	*Moods or feelings?*	*Thoughts then?*	*Thoughts now?*

Day 4 Experience?	Sensations, in detail?	Moods or feelings?	Thoughts then?	Thoughts now?

The doing mode of mind controls what we habitually look out for—in a depressed mind-state we focus on the negative and what's wrong, in an anxious mind-state we focus on what's threatening or dangerous, and so on for other kinds of doing modes of mind. Deliberately looking out for pleasant experiences can retune our attention and open us to the many small delights of life that were always there but that we never noticed—the reflections of trees on water, the laughter of children, the flowers by the side of the road. . . .

Day 5 Experience?	Sensations, in detail?	Moods or feelings?	Thoughts then?	Thoughts now?

Day 6 Experience?	Sensations, in detail?	Moods or feelings?	Thoughts then?	Thoughts now?

At the end of the week, take a moment to reflect on your experience with the Pleasant Experiences Calendar.

Write here **one thing worth remembering** that you learned or noticed:

_____

_____

_____

_____

_____

_____

_____

_____

_____

_____

Dreaming the Real

I'm lying down looking at the colour
of sky falling through trees, dreaming
the real, tasting what it feels like to love it.

Why did it take me so long to let go, simply
exhale, so the day could breathe itself in
and open without me standing in the way?

How could I forget the grace of my own body
strong as this blue, tender as the white
of the wild blossom, warm as midday light?

Let me practise a patience bold enough
to hold every weather, trusting the elements,
the beauty of rain, all its shades of grey.

I want whatever's real to be enough. At least
it's a place to begin. And to master the art
of loving it; feel it love me back under my skin.

LINDA FRANCE

7

Week 3:
Coming Home to the Present
GATHERING THE SCATTERED MIND

Orientation

Try this very brief experiment:

1. After you've read these instructions, put down the book and make a note of the time on your watch or on a clock.
2. Sit without doing anything for a minute.
3. At the end of the minute, pick up the book and go back to reading.

Where was your mind in that minute? Was it right here in this room, fully engaged with the ever-present now as it unfolded from one moment to the next?

Or did your mind take you far away from this time and place? Perhaps it took you forward to the future, to events coming up in a few minutes, hours, weeks, or years. Or maybe it took you back to the past—to events that happened earlier today, yesterday, last week, or years ago.

If your experience was any of these, you've just engaged in **mental time travel**—the third of the seven core features of the doing mode of mind (page 17).

Our capacity to travel to different times and places in our minds, when used consciously and knowingly, allows us to plan for the future and learn from the past.

But when the driven–doing mode of mind whisks us away from the here and now without our knowledge or consent, we have problems:

- Rumination about the past drags us back into depression or anger.
- Worry about the future tips us into anxiety.
- Anticipating everything we "have to" do makes us feel burdened, exhausted, and stressed out.

In Week 3 we explore how, wherever we are, whatever we are doing, we can learn to disengage from unhelpful and unintended mental time travel:

1. by using the breath as an ever-present anchor to return to the here and now
2. through mindful awareness of the body in movement
3. with a mini-meditation—the 3-Minute Breathing Space

With practice, we can learn how to gather and settle our scattered minds. We then experience the calm and peace that awaits us beneath the turmoil of the driven-thinking mind.

Daily Practice

During Week 3, practice each of these exercises **for 6 out of the next 7 days:***

1. Combined Stretch and Breath Meditation (days 1, 3, 5)
2. Mindful Movement Meditation (days 2, 4, 6)
3. 3-Minute Breathing Space
4. Unpleasant Experiences Calendar

Taking Good Care of Your Body

Two of the practices this week involve some gentle physical exercise.

The intention of these practices is to become aware of physical sensations and feelings throughout your body, honoring and investigating the limitations of your body, and letting go of any tendency to push beyond your limits.

If you have any back or other health difficulties that may cause problems, make your own decision as to which (if any) of these exercises to do and consult your physician or physical therapist if you are unsure.

---

*The first two practices are scheduled for alternate days—so, although it may seem that there are more practice and instructions this week, it actually works out much the same as usual.

1. Combined Stretch and Breath Meditation

On Days 1, 3, and 5, set up whatever you need for sitting meditation practice—a chair, cushion, or meditation bench—and then follow the instructions on audio track 6 (*Stretch and Breath Meditation*). This practice involves a few minutes of guided mindful stretching followed immediately by a sitting meditation.

The mindful stretching involves a series of gentle standing stretches—please remember to take good care of your body. If you have any problems with your back or other health difficulties, first listen to the instructions without following them and then think carefully about whether you should do all or any of the practices described. Feel free to skip those that may be too difficult at this time and simply imagine yourself doing them along with the instructions.

A summary of the instructions appears on pages 88–89.

STRETCH AND BREATH MEDITATION: MINDFUL STRETCHING

1. First, find a place where you can stand in bare feet or socks with your feet about hip width apart, with your knees unlocked so that your legs can bend slightly and with your feet parallel (it's actually unusual to stand with your feet like this, and this, itself, can generate some novel bodily sensations).

2. Next, remind yourself of the intention of this practice: to become aware, as best you can, of physical sensations and feelings throughout the body as you engage in a series of gentle stretches, honoring and investigating the limitations of your body in every moment, as best you can letting go of any tendency to push beyond your limits or to compete with either yourself or others.

3. Then, on an inbreath, slowly and mindfully raise your arms out to the sides, raising them, slowly and mindfully, until your hands are above your head; as you do this, feel the tension in the muscles as they work to lift the arms and then maintain them in the stretch.

4. Then, letting the breath move in and out freely at its own pace, continue to stretch upward, your fingertips gently pushing toward the sky, your feet firmly grounded on the floor, feeling the stretch in the muscles and joints of the body all the way from your feet and legs up through your back, shoulders, into your arms and hands and fingers.

5. Maintain that stretch for a time, breathing freely in and out, noticing any changes in the sensations and feelings in your body with the breath and as you continue to hold the stretch. Of course, this might include a sense of increasing tension or discomfort, and if so, see if it's possible to open to that as well.

6. Then, when you are ready, slowly, very slowly, on an outbreath, allow your

arms to come back down. Lower them slowly, with the wrists bent so that the fingers point upward and the palms are pushing outward (again, an unusual position) until your arms come back to rest along your sides, hanging from the shoulders.

7. Allow your eyes to close gently and focus attention on the movements of the breath and the sensations and feelings throughout your body as you stand here, perhaps noticing the contrast in the physical sense of release (and often relief) associated with returning to a neutral stance.

8. Continue now by mindfully stretching each arm and hand up in turn, as if you were picking fruit from a tree that is just out of reach, with full awareness of the sensations throughout your body and of your breath. See what happens to the extension of your hand and to the breath if you lift the opposite heel off the floor while stretching up.

9. Next, slowly and mindfully raise both arms up high, keeping them parallel to each other, and then allow your body to bend over as a whole to the left, forming a big curve that extends sideways from your feet right through your torso, arms, and hands and fingers. Then, on an inbreath, come back to the center, and on the outbreath, slowly bend over, forming a curve in the opposite direction. And now, returning to a central standing position, allow your arms to come down slowly until they are hanging loosely alongside the body.

10. Now you can play with rolling your shoulders while letting your arms dangle passively. First, raise your shoulders upward toward your ears as far as they will go; then backward as if you were attempting to draw your shoulder blades together; then let them drop back down; then squeeze your shoulders together in front of your body as far as they will go, as if you were trying to touch them together, with your arms passive and dangling. Continue "rolling" through these various positions as smoothly and mindfully as you can, with your arms dangling all the while, first in one direction and then in the opposite direction, in a forward and backward "rowing" motion.

11. Then, once you have rested in a neutral standing posture again, play with slowly and mindfully rolling your head around in a semi-circle. First of all, moving the chin down towards the chest, letting it hang here, but not forcing it at all . . . and then moving the head over to the left-hand side so the left ear comes down toward the left shoulder. Then slowly moving the head over to the other side so the right ear comes toward the right shoulder, . . . and then moving the head down toward the chest again . . . then when you are ready, reversing the direction of the movement.

12. And finally, at the end of this sequence of movements, remain still for a while, in a standing posture, and tune in to the sensations from your body and the effects of these stretches, before moving to a sitting meditation.

Mindful Standing Stretches

Steps 1–2   Steps 3–5   Steps 6–7   Step 8   Step 9

BOTH SIDES

BOTH SIDES

Step 10

Step 11

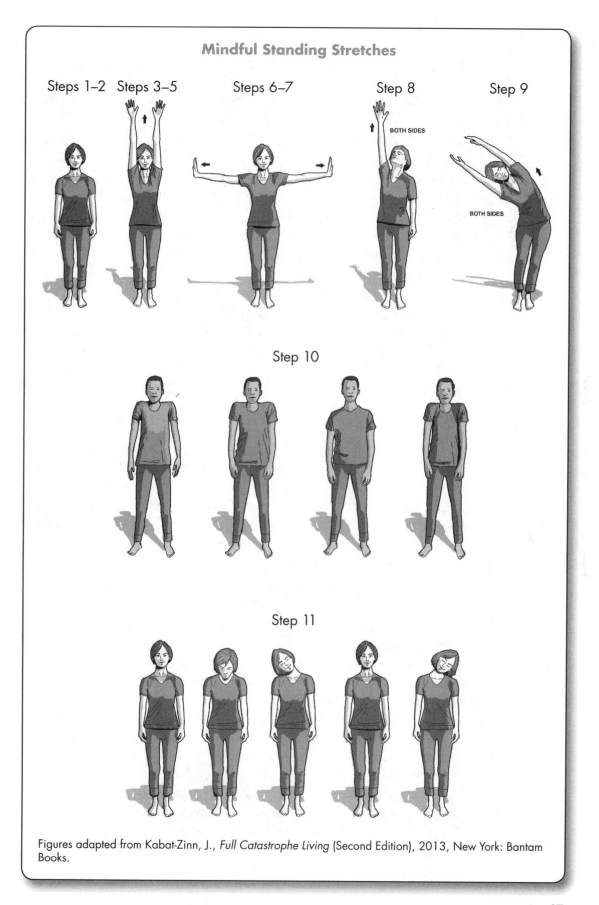

Figures adapted from Kabat-Zinn, J., *Full Catastrophe Living* (Second Edition), 2013, New York: Bantam Books.

STRETCH AND BREATH MEDITATION: SITTING MEDITATION

1. Practice mindfulness of the breath, as described earlier (page 73), for 10 minutes.

2. Then, when you feel reasonably settled on awareness of the breath, intentionally allow the awareness to expand around the breath to include, as well, a sense of physical sensations throughout your whole body. While still aware, in the background, of the movements of the breath in your lower abdomen, let the primary focus for your awareness be a sense of your body as a whole and the changing patterns of sensation throughout your body. You may find that you get a sense of the movements of the breath throughout your body, as if your whole body were breathing.

3. Within this wider sense of the body and breath, notice the patterns of physical sensations that arise where the body makes contact with the floor, chair, cushion, or bench—the sensations of touch, pressure, or contact of your feet or knees with the floor; your buttocks with whatever supports them; your hands where they rest on each other or on your thighs. As best you can, hold all these sensations, together with the sense of the breath and of your body as a whole, in a wider space of awareness.

4. Your mind will wander repeatedly away from the breath and body sensations—this is natural, to be expected, and in no way a mistake or a failure. Whenever you notice that your awareness has drifted away from the sense of your body or breath, you might want to congratulate yourself; you have "woken up." Gently note where your mind was (some people find it helpful to say "thinking" very lightly to themselves at the back of their mind), and then, as kindly as you can, refocus your attention back to the breathing and to a sense of your body as a whole.

5. As best you can, keep things simple, gently attending to the actuality of sensations throughout your body from one moment to the next.

6. As you sit, some sensations may be particularly intense, such as pains in the back or knees or shoulders. You may find that awareness is repeatedly drawn to these sensations and away from your intended focus on your breath or body as a whole. You may want to use these times to experiment with choosing either to intentionally shift posture or to remain still and bring the focus of awareness right into the region of intensity. If you choose to remain still, then, as best you can, explore with gentle attention the detailed pattern of sensations here: What, precisely, do the sensations feel like? Where exactly are they? Do they vary over time or from one part of the region of intensity to another? See if it's possible to just *feel* them, rather than *think* about them. You may want to use the breath as a way to carry awareness into such regions of intensity, "breathing in" to them, just as in the body scan; and on the outbreath, "breathing out" from those sensations, softening and opening as the breath leaves.

7. Whenever you find yourself "carried away" from awareness in the moment by the intensity of physical sensations, or in any other way, remind yourself that you can always reconnect with the here and now by refocusing awareness on the movements of the breath or on a sense of your body as a whole. Once you have **re-gathered** yourself in this way, you can allow the awareness to expand once more to include a sense of sensations throughout your body.

8. And in the closing minutes of this sitting, bring your attention back to focus on your breathing in the abdomen, tuning in to any and all sensations on each inbreath and each outbreath. And as you sit here and as you breathe, allow yourself to cultivate a sense of moment-to-moment awareness, remembering that the breath is available to you at any moment of your day, to allow you to feel grounded, to give you a sense of balance, and to accept yourself just as you are in each moment.

Day 1 (Stretch and Breath): In the sitting part of the meditation, what did you do when you noticed that your mind had wandered?

_____

_____

_____

_____

_____

I have been thinking of a thousand and one other things. It's very difficult to keep myself from going into the future, thinking about things. I try to control it, and maybe it works for 2 minutes, but then I go off again.

It's natural to feel we should do something to control or get rid of thoughts, so it's important to remember that we are not aiming to push thoughts away or squash them down—if we do that, we just give them more energy and they bounce back even more strongly.

We are not aiming to put the brakes on the thinking mind— the aim is to recognize "Here is thinking," and, as best we can, let go of the thinking and focus back on the breath.

Day 3 (Stretch and Breath): In the sitting part of the meditation, how kind or unkind were you to yourself when you noticed the mind wandering again and again?

_____

_____

_____

_____

_____

I felt annoyed with myself—it's such a simple thing, I should be able to do it. I'm sure other people don't have this problem—I must try harder.

Most people at this stage of the program spend a good deal of time struggling to maintain the focus of their attention on the breath. As best you can, acknowledge the wandering of the mind as "just how it is right now" and respond with as much gentleness, kindness, and humor as you can—and if you can't be kind, be kind to that too!

Day 5 (Stretch and Breath): In the sitting part of the meditation, how much physical discomfort did you experience? How did you respond?

_____

_____

_____

_____

_____

My back was aching, my knees were painful—it took a real effort to stay focused on the breath and not move—but I hung in there until the end.

The idea isn't to feel you have to endure physical pain indefinitely as a test of endurance or character! It's best not to move as soon as you feel any hint of discomfort (because that will strengthen the habit of automatic avoidance) but, once you've explored the intense sensations with wise and gentle awareness, it's fine to move mindfully as an act of kindness to yourself.

Hurray for Mind Wandering!

Mind wandering is not a mistake or a failure—it is just what minds do.

The aim of this practice is not to prevent your mind from wandering but to use the times when you notice that the mind has wandered to develop your skills of:

1. **recognizing** that this has happened—**without giving yourself a hard time**
2. **pausing** long enough to know where your mind is in that moment
3. **letting go** of what was on your mind
4. **gently and kindly** bringing your attention back to the breath

The practice gives us chance after chance after chance to come back from mental time travel and begin again, in this moment, with this breath.

Noticing when the mind has wandered and bringing it back is the core of meditation practice—that's how we learn to know when we are in doing mode and gently release ourselves and enter being mode.

2. Mindful Movement Meditation

On Days 2, 4, and 6 this week, play audio track 5 (*Mindful Movement*) and follow the instructions as best you can. Sketches of the mindful movement postures are shown on pages 92–95. (It's not easy to do mindful movement from written instructions, so we haven't provided any; please use the audio instructions.)

This practice involves a series of gentle body stretches. Once again, please remember to **take good care of your body**. If you have any problems with your back or other health difficulties, feel free to listen to the instructions first without following them and then think carefully about whether you should do all or any of the practices described. As you are guided through the practice, let the wisdom of your own body decide which stretch to do and for how long.

The intention of this practice is to help you tune in to sensations in the body just as they are. It's not about getting fit or challenging yourself to stretch farther than you've done before. **See if it's possible to stretch without striving.**

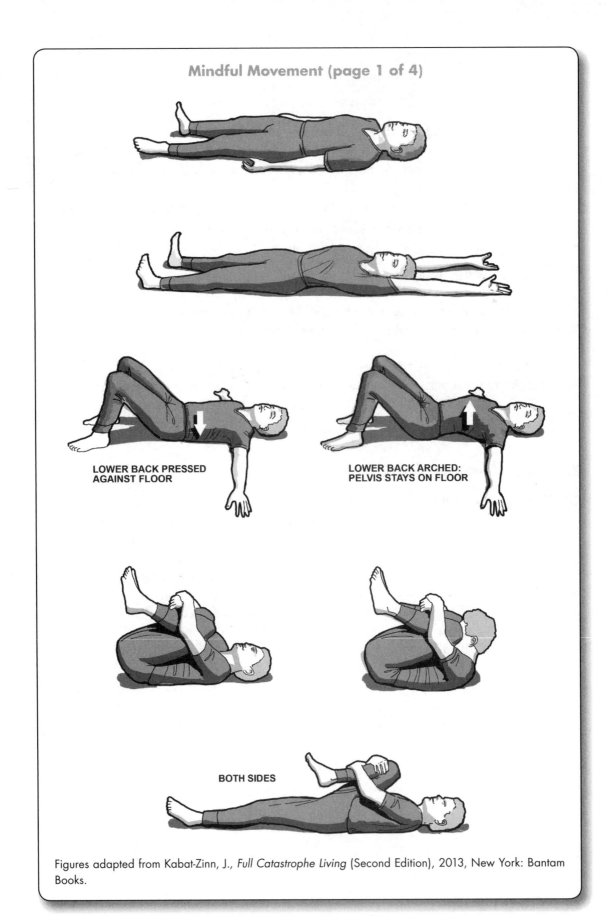

LOWER BACK PRESSED AGAINST FLOOR

LOWER BACK ARCHED: PELVIS STAYS ON FLOOR

BOTH SIDES

Figures adapted from Kabat-Zinn, J., *Full Catastrophe Living* (Second Edition), 2013, New York: Bantam Books.

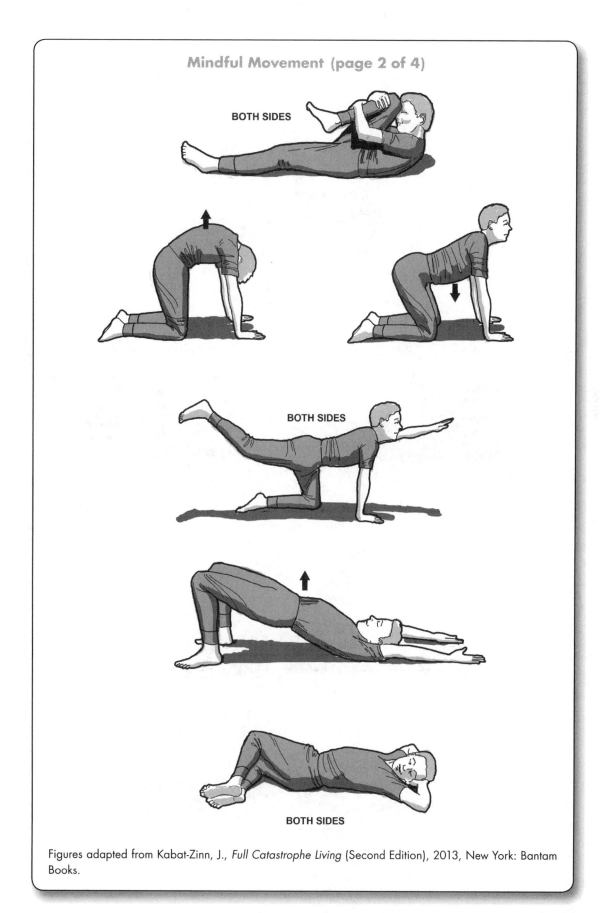

Figures adapted from Kabat-Zinn, J., *Full Catastrophe Living* (Second Edition), 2013, New York: Bantam Books.

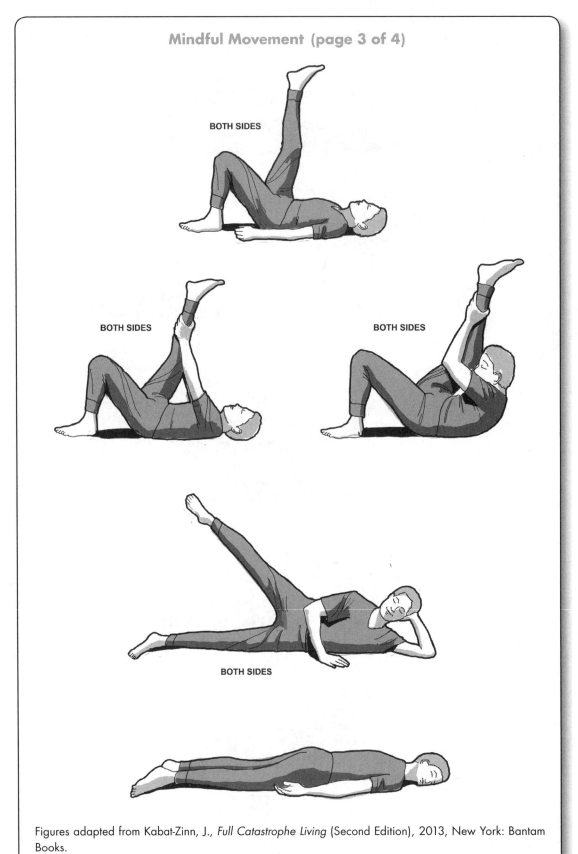

BOTH SIDES

BOTH SIDES

BOTH SIDES

BOTH SIDES

Figures adapted from Kabat-Zinn, J., *Full Catastrophe Living* (Second Edition), 2013, New York: Bantam Books.

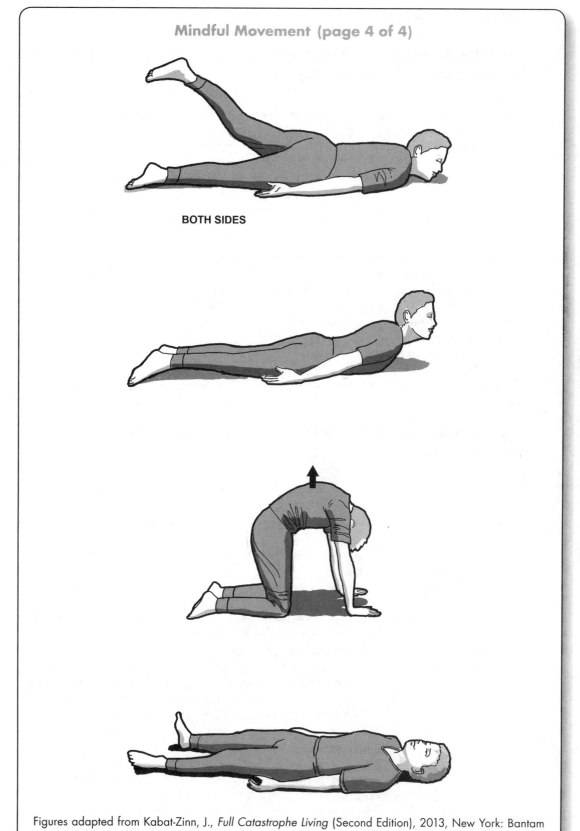

BOTH SIDES

Figures adapted from Kabat-Zinn, J., *Full Catastrophe Living* (Second Edition), 2013, New York: Bantam Books.

Day 2 (Mindful Movement): How easy was it to be aware of body sensations in this practice, compared to the sitting meditation?

_____

_____

_____

_____

_____

> For me this was easier—the sensations from the body as I moved and stretched were much "louder" and easier to notice than when I was sitting—and because there was less silence, my mind didn't wander so far away. I enjoyed the practice!

> Many people find the same—that's why mindfulness of the body in movement, wherever we are, can be such a helpful way to gather the scattered mind and return to the here and now.

Day 4 (Mindful Movement): How did you respond to any intense body sensations you experienced?

_____

_____

_____

_____

> I didn't want to feel them! So I didn't really push or stretch myself as much as I should.

> The skill of _directly approaching and moving the awareness right into unpleasant body sensations_ is a central part of learning to work with difficult emotions _in the body_. Mindful stretching allows us to "work the edge" with intense body sensations—we gently move awareness closer and closer to intense sensations until we choose to go no further, backing off a little if we like, and then, when we are ready, we gradually approach the intensity once more, knowing we can choose to ease the stretch at any point.

By intentionally moving our awareness gently and gradually *toward* uncomfortable sensations we begin to undo the deeply rooted habit of needing to avoid unpleasant feelings— which is the energy that keeps *all* difficult emotions going.

Day 6 (Mindful Movement): What *bodily* reactions to intense sensations did you notice? How did those reactions feel?

_____

_____

_____

_____

I noticed I was tensing and bracing against the stretches—and that, itself, felt uncomfortable.

This practice can help us begin to see the way we often ADD EXTRA to unpleasant sensations or feelings— there is (a) the unavoidable discomfort from holding a stretch longer than usual and (b) the <u>avoidable</u> discomfort from <u>resisting</u> those sensations or from <u>striving</u> and <u>pushing ourselves</u> to reach a standard that WE (not the instructions!) have set for how the practice <u>should</u> be done.

We will have much more to say next week about how we habitually ADD EXTRA to unpleasant sensations or feelings.

3. The 3-Minute Breathing Space

The aim of MBCT is to use mindfulness as a way to gather the scattered mind and relate more skillfully to difficult emotions as they arise, wherever you are.

In most situations it's not possible to close your eyes and meditate for 40 minutes!

To bridge the gap between extended "formal" meditation practice (body scan, sitting meditation, mindful movement) and everyday life where you actually need to use mindfulness skills, we use a mini-meditation—the 3-Minute Breathing Space.

To begin, we embed this practice in the routine of each day of your life.

Every day this week, take a 3-minute breathing space **three times a day** at times you have chosen in advance—it's best if you can aim for the same times each day.

Once a day, use audio track 8 (*3-Minute Breathing Space*) for guidance for the breathing space. At the other times, guide yourself from memory or using the instructions below.

Keep track of daily practice of these **R**EGULAR breathing spaces on your smart phone or on a card you carry around with you, then record them at the end of the day by circling an R here:

Day 1: **R**   **R**   **R**   Day 2: **R**   **R**   **R**   Day 3: **R**   **R**   **R**

Day 4: **R**   **R**   **R**   Day 5: **R**   **R**   **R**   Day 6: **R**   **R**   **R**

3-MINUTE BREATHING SPACE INSTRUCTIONS

Preparation

Begin by deliberately adopting an erect and dignified posture, whether you are sitting or standing. If possible, close your eyes. Then take about 1 minute to guide yourself through each of the following three steps:

Step 1. Becoming Aware

Bringing your awareness to your inner experience, ask: **What is my experience *right now*?**

- What *thoughts* are going through your mind? As best you can, acknowledge thoughts as mental events, perhaps putting them into words.
- What *feelings* are here? Turn toward any sense of emotional discomfort or unpleasant feelings, acknowledging their presence.
- What *body sensations* are here right now? Perhaps quickly scan your body to pick up any sensations of tightness or bracing.

Step 2. Gathering

Now redirect your attention to focus on the physical sensations of the breath breathing itself.

Move in close to the sense of the breath in the abdomen . . . feeling the sensations of the abdominal wall expanding as the breath comes in . . . and falling back as the breath goes out.

Follow the breath all the way in and all the way out, using the breathing to anchor yourself in the present. If your mind wanders away at any time, gently escort it back to the breath.

Step 3. Expanding

Now expand the field of your awareness around your breathing so that it includes a sense of the body as a whole, your posture, and facial expression.

If you become aware of any sensations of discomfort, tension, or resistance, take your awareness there by breathing into them on the inbreath. Then breathe out from those sensations, softening and opening with the outbreath.

As best you can, bring this expanded awareness to the next moments of your day.

The breathing space is THE way to step out of automatic pilot and reconnect with the present moment.

When should I do my three breathing spaces each day?

It's best to choose times that are linked to events that are already firm fixtures in your daily routine. For example, you might take a breathing space as soon as you get out of bed, or just before you shower, after you have eaten breakfast, lunch, or dinner, when you take a regular break at work, on the train or bus as you go to or from work, or just before you get ready for bed—see if you can find the times that work best for you.

Make a note here of the three times at which you plan to take a Regular Breathing Space each day:

Time 1 _____

Time 2 _____

Time 3 _____

The 3-minute breathing space is the single most important practice in the MBCT program.

Why don't we just go straight to Step 2—gathering attention on the breath? Isn't that the key skill we're learning? What's the point of Steps 1 and 3?

Learning to switch attention to the breath is a very useful way to step out of rumination, worry, obsessive planning, etc. But if that's all we did, we'd just be changing WHAT the mind is working on, rather than HOW it's working—most likely we'd still be in doing mode. Steps 1 and 3 are there to help us shift to being mode—to change HOW the mind is working as well as WHAT it is working on.

So what happens in Step 1?

In Step 1 we bring thoughts, feelings, and body sensations into the scope of conscious rather than automatic processing. By deliberately bringing an interested awareness to our inner experience, even if it is difficult or unpleasant, we strengthen the approach tendencies of the mind and weaken the tendency to avoid. We also do our best to see thoughts, feelings, and sensations for what they are—just events passing through the mind, rather than realities or infallible messages that something is wrong.

And in Step 3?

In Step 3, having gathered and settled the mind as best we can, we expand our awareness so that we can include all our experience of the body in that moment (not just the breath) in the scope of being mode. In that way, we have prepared the mind so that we can greet all life experience in being mode as we exit the 3-minute breathing space and reconnect with our day. And, if there are difficult or unpleasant experiences around, we have already prepared ourselves to receive them with openness and acceptance by deliberately cultivating a gentler attitude to any discomfort we experience in the body in Step 3.

The breathing space sets us up to encounter life in a different frame of mind, coming fully home to the present, rather than just giving ourselves a break from thinking.

4. Unpleasant Experiences Calendar

Each day, aim to be aware of one unpleasant experience **as it is happening**.

It doesn't have to be anything extreme—just an experience that felt unpleasant, unwanted, or irksome in some way. It might be as slight as some passing mild irritation or sense of weariness.

As with last week, this practice invites you to make a conscious effort to pay attention differently—to deliberately turn **toward** the unpleasant experience (not necessarily our usual response) and to see if it is possible to become aware of the separate aspects of the experience—the unpleasant feeling itself, any other feelings around, any thoughts going through your mind, and the sensations in your body.

Separating the unpleasant experience into its components in this way is a pivotal step in beginning to learn a new and more skillful way to relate to unpleasant emotions and situations.

See if you can be aware of the difference between, on the one hand, the *unpleasant feelings* themselves and, on the other hand, any *reaction* to unpleasantness.

Use the following questions to focus your awareness on the details of the experience as it is happening. You can write it down later.

What was the experience?	What sensations did you feel in your body, in detail?	What moods or feelings did you notice?	What thoughts went through your mind?	What thoughts are in your mind now as you write this down?
Example: Waiting for the cable company to come out and fix our line. Realize that I am missing an important meeting at work.	Temples throbbing, tightness in my neck and shoulders, pacing back and forth	Angry, helpless	"Is this what they mean by service?" "This is one meeting I didn't want to miss."	I hope I don't have to go through that again soon.

Write down your thoughts word for word if that's how you experience them, or describe any images in your mind's eye; note exactly where any sensations were felt in the body and what they were. Use the act of recording itself as an opportunity to become aware of any thoughts going through your mind as you write.

Day 1 *What was the experience?*	*What sensations did you feel in your body, in detail?*	*What moods or feelings did you notice?*	*What thoughts went through your mind?*	*What thoughts are in your mind now as you write this down?*

We have an automatic tendency to react to unpleasant feelings by wanting to get rid of them or get away from them. This "not wanting" or "aversion" itself feels unpleasant. If we look carefully, over time we may recognize the difference between unpleasant feelings and the reaction of "not wanting" or pushing away. The body can give us clues—you may have noticed tension, contraction, or resistance in the body linked to "not wanting." Each of us has our own pattern of sensations—perhaps in the face, shoulders, belly, hands, or chest—look out for your particular pattern.

Day 2 Experience?	Sensations, in detail?	Moods or feelings?	Thoughts then?	Thoughts now?

Not wanting to experience unpleasant feelings means we try to keep difficult or uncomfortable experiences at a distance—we don't look closely at them. This means they can seem like vaguely threatening "big bad blobs."

Notice carefully what happens when you "de-blob" unpleasant experiences by focusing attention closely on them—homing in on their separate components—body sensations, feelings, and thoughts.

Day 3 Experience?	Sensations, in detail?	Moods or feelings?	Thoughts then?	Thoughts now?

Day 4 Experience?	Sensations, in detail?	Moods or feelings?	Thoughts then?	Thoughts now?

Often it's the stories we tell ourselves about our unpleasant experiences—the thoughts that get triggered by them—that create and sustain the suffering we experience. For example, we might tell ourselves, "I shouldn't be feeling like this. Why am I so stupid and weak?" Or we might ask, "What if this keeps on happening?" And then we just feel even worse.

See if it is possible to notice the ways that your thinking can feed the vicious cycles that increase unhappiness.

Day 5 Experience?	Sensations, in detail?	Moods or feelings?	Thoughts then?	Thoughts now?

Day 6 Experience?	Sensations, in detail?	Moods or feelings?	Thoughts then?	Thoughts now?

At the end of the week, take a moment to reflect on your experience with the Unpleasant Experiences Calendar. Note here **one thing worth remembering** that you learned or noticed:

_____

_____

_____

_____

_____

_____

_____

_____

Thank you for giving **the daily practice for Week 3** your best efforts and intentions.

The Peace of Wild Things

When despair for the world grows in me
and I wake in the night at the least sound
in fear of what my life and my children's lives may be,
I go and lie down where the wood drake
rests in his beauty on the water, and the great heron feeds.
I come into the peace of wild things
who do not tax their lives with forethought
of grief. I come into the presence of still water.
And I feel above me the day-blind stars
waiting with their light. For a time
I rest in the grace of the world, and am free.

WENDELL BERRY

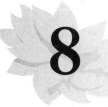

8

Week 4:
Recognizing Aversion

Orientation

We can react to unpleasant and uncomfortable feelings in many different ways.

Jake: "This morning I noticed a sense of sadness arising. I gritted my teeth and forced myself to carry on regardless. I could feel my whole body braced against the feeling." ☐

Rose: "When I get anxious, I go over and over possible disasters and difficulties ('what if . . . what if . . . what if?'), trying to find ways to stay in control." ☐

Vince: "Yesterday it came to me how much of the time I don't want to be feeling what I'm feeling. I just seem to sort of tune out." ☐

Maria: "When I start to feel low or blue, my mind drags up things that have happened that might explain why I'm feeling that way; I end up going over and over the past—what did I do wrong? What did I say wrong? What's wrong with me that I feel this way?" ☐

Jean: "My bus was late today. I got really angry with the stupidity of the bus company for their poor organization—then I was angry with myself for letting a little thing like that upset me so much." ☐

Anne-Marie: "This afternoon my boss criticized a report I had prepared. I became really agitated—I felt so much pressure to do <u>something</u> that I was hardly aware of what I was doing." ☐

Do any of these remind you of anything? Take a moment to reflect on what **you** do when things go wrong or you are faced with unpleasant or difficult feelings. You may find it helpful to think back to what you noticed with the Unpleasant Experiences Calendar last week. Check off any of the boxes on page 107 that echo your own experience.

On the surface, the reactions of Jake, Rose, Maria, Vince, Anne-Marie, and Jean may look quite different. But deep down they are all driven by the same underlying need to avoid actually experiencing unpleasant or painful feelings.

This deeply ingrained habit, which we all share, is called **aversion**.

Aversion is the drive to avoid, escape, get rid of,
numb out from, or destroy things
we experience as unpleasant.

It is the power behind the driven-doing
that keeps us entangled in negative emotions
such as depression, anxiety, anger, and stress.

Freeze-Framing Aversion

If you carefully investigate how you relate to unpleasant feelings, you will see that there are two crucial steps:

Step 1: an unpleasant feeling arises;

Step 2: your mind reacts to the unpleasant feeling by trying, in one way or another, to avoid experiencing the feeling or the thing that caused the feeling.

These two steps played out with Jake, Rose, Maria, Vince, Anne-Marie, and Jean like this:

	Step 1	Step 2
Jake	Sad feeling	Resistance
Rose	Anxious feeling	Worry
Maria	Feeling low	Rumination
Vince	Most feelings	Tuning out
Anne-Marie	Feeling criticized	"Have to do something"
Jean	Angry feeling	Self-criticism

Most often Steps 1 and 2 get rolled together: we don't see them as separate and different; we just feel bad.

By becoming more closely acquainted with this 1–2 pattern you can take a powerful step toward freeing yourself from emotional pain.

Why? Even if you can't do much about Step 1—the arising of the unpleasant feeling—with mindfulness, you can always do something about Step 2; **you can release the lock-nut of aversion that keeps you tied to feelings you don't want**.

A central aim of this week's practice is to begin to unlearn the habit of avoiding and disconnecting from unpleasant experiences. The way to do that is to become an expert in how aversion affects **you**.

> Deliberately turning to face, investigate, and recognize unpleasant feelings—and your reactions to them—is a powerful affirmation that you do not *have* to get rid of them. Instead they can be held in awareness, seen for what they are, and met with *conscious response* rather than *automatic reaction*.

Isn't aversion natural? Doesn't it make sense to want to get rid of or avoid things that are unpleasant?

Yes, it's very natural. Earlier in evolution, when the dangerous things we encountered were in the <u>outside</u> world (saber-tooth tigers, human enemies, forest fires, etc.), aversion literally saved our lives. That's why it's hard-wired, deep inside us.

The problem comes when the unpleasant and difficult things are in the <u>inside</u> world—when the "enemies" are our own oppressive and threatening thoughts, feelings, emotions, and sense of self. None of us can run fast enough to escape these inner experiences—and we can't get rid of them by fighting them or trying to destroy them.

But how does aversion toward our inner experience make things WORSE?

First, aversion itself feels unpleasant. It's meant to—that's why we want to get rid of the thing that's creating it. But when that thing is itself an unpleasant feeling, aversion just adds to the total sum of unpleasantness around—we feel worse, not better.

Second, trying to get rid of unpleasant thoughts and feelings through an effort of will just keeps us stuck to them even more firmly—the more we push them away, the harder they push back, and we end up exhausting ourselves and creating ever more unpleasant feelings.

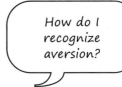

How do I recognize aversion?

Aversion takes different forms from one person to another. Mostly, it involves: (1) An overall feeling of "not wanting"—not wanting things to be as they are, not wanting to be having the experiences we are having, not wanting to be the person we think we are—one way or another we feel we <u>need</u> things to be different. This will, itself, feel unpleasant. (2) A characteristic pattern of sensations in the body—often a sense of pushing away, contraction, resistance, tightness, bracing, or intensity. Some people experience tension in the face or forehead. Others feel their shoulders braced in resistance, or a sense of contraction or intensity in the abdomen or chest. Their hands may be clenched. All these sensations, themselves, feel unpleasant.

In the practice this week you are invited to continue the exploration of your own pattern of bodily reactions to unpleasant experiences that you began with the Unpleasant Experiences Calendar last week.

Seeing Negative Thoughts with Less Aversion

When we first developed MBCT, our main focus was on helping people who had been depressed in the past. We used this next exercise because the questionnaire had been developed with depression in mind. But in teaching MBCT more widely we've discovered that almost everyone recognizes some of these thoughts when life gets overwhelming. We'll describe the exercise as we did it originally. If your main problem isn't depression, you might, nonetheless, like to see how relevant it is to you.

If you have experienced deep depression in the past, think back to a time when you were at your most depressed. On the facing page are some of the thoughts that can come to mind at such times. Put an X in column A next to each thought that you recognize as one you've experienced when depressed.

CHECKLIST OF NEGATIVE THOUGHTS

	A	B	C
1. I feel like I'm up against the world.	_____	_____	_____
2. I'm no good.	_____	_____	_____
3. Why can't I ever succeed?	_____	_____	_____
4. No one understands me.	_____	_____	_____
5. I've let people down.	_____	_____	_____
6. I don't think I can go on.	_____	_____	_____
7. I wish I were a better person.	_____	_____	_____
8. I'm so weak.	_____	_____	_____
9. My life's not going the way I want it to.	_____	_____	_____
10. I'm so disappointed in myself.	_____	_____	_____
11. Nothing feels good anymore.	_____	_____	_____
12. I can't stand this anymore.	_____	_____	_____
13. I can't get started.	_____	_____	_____
14. What's wrong with me?	_____	_____	_____
15. I wish I were somewhere else.	_____	_____	_____
16. I can't get things together.	_____	_____	_____
17. I hate myself.	_____	_____	_____
18. I'm worthless.	_____	_____	_____
19. I wish I could just disappear.	_____	_____	_____
20. What's the matter with me?	_____	_____	_____
21. I'm a loser.	_____	_____	_____
22. My life is a mess.	_____	_____	_____
23. I'm a failure.	_____	_____	_____
24. I'll never make it.	_____	_____	_____
25. I feel so helpless.	_____	_____	_____
26. Something has to change.	_____	_____	_____
27. There must be something wrong with me.	_____	_____	_____
28. My future is bleak.	_____	_____	_____
29. It's just not worth it.	_____	_____	_____
30. I can't finish anything.	_____	_____	_____

Now, for each of the thoughts with an X in column A, go back and rate how much you believed it **when you were at your most depressed**—give it a score in column B from 0 (you didn't believe it at all) to 10 (you believed it 100%). It may be difficult to remember this clearly, but do the best you can.

Next, think back to a time **when you were not feeling depressed at all** and rate how much you believed each thought then by giving it a score from 0 to 10 in column C.

Finally, take a look at the scores you've given in columns B and C and jot down what you notice and any reflections here:

_____

_____

_____

_____

_____

Here are some comments from participants in an MBCT class for depression:

Anya: *"I recognized nearly all the thoughts! When I was depressed, I believed them 100%—but now hardly at all."*

Carlos: *"Me too! When I was really down, I thought, That's just how it is. Now I ask myself, What was all that about? How could I ever have believed all that stuff?"*

Tina: *"Why has no one shown me this before? If doctors know about this, why didn't they tell me? It would have shown they understood how I felt. I thought it was me—I was tired, things were getting me down. . . . Now I realize it's depression. If only someone had told me sooner, it would have saved me so much pain."*

From our experience with using this exercise with hundreds of women and men who have been clinically depressed, two things stand out:

1. Most people who have been depressed recognize having had some, if not all, of the negative thoughts on the list.

2. Belief in the thoughts changes dramatically with mood. When people are depressed, they believe the thoughts unquestioningly, but when they feel better they believe the thoughts much less, if at all.

Do you recognize anything similar in your own experience?

The fact that most people who get clinically depressed have very similar negative thoughts tells us something very important: **these thoughts are features of the depressed state, not us.**

When we feel low, these thoughts often feel like the truth about us. But in fact they are symptoms of depression—just as a high temperature is a symptom of flu.

That's why belief in these thoughts can change so much as mood changes. Because the negative thoughts are reflections of an underlying depressed state of mind, or mood—rather than accurate reflections of the truth about us—belief in the thoughts changes as the state of mind that gave birth to them comes and goes.

When we can see the negative thoughts and feelings of depression for what they really are—symptoms rather than "me" or the truth—we don't need to take them so personally **and we are less likely to react with aversion.**

> What about other states of mind—like anxiety, anger, or being stressed out?

> What's true of depression is true of them too. Imagine you are someone who worries about what people think of you. You have to make an important presentation to colleagues. While the presentation is still a long way in the future, you can shrug off negative thoughts about the talk. But, as the day approaches, you get more and more anxious, and your worries become more and more convincing. On the day itself, you are absolutely sure something dreadful will happen. You give the talk, it goes fine, you relax and look back on your worries and predictions of catastrophe and think, "What on earth was all that about?"

It's quite likely that focusing on negative thoughts and thinking back to times when things were very bad for you may have made you feel low or sad. If that's true, now might be a good time to

Take a breathing space.

Seeing Negative States of Mind with Less Aversion

It's not just negative thoughts that we take personally and react to with aversion.

We react to the negative states of mind from which the thoughts arise in just the same way.

If you have been depressed, have you ever blamed yourself for being lazy because you have no energy? Or perhaps you felt guilty and selfish when you noticed that you were no longer interested in making time to be with friends or family. Perhaps you labeled yourself stupid because you couldn't concentrate or because you seemed to have slowed down so much?

What if these are not signs of personal failing or inadequacy?

What if they are actually symptoms of depression?

Throughout the world, psychiatrists and psychologists use the presence of a number of core features to make a diagnosis of depression. These features include being tired and apathetic, no longer interested in the events and activities you once enjoyed, and having a hard time making decisions or concentrating (for example, on tasks at work or watching TV at home), along with feeling sad, worthless, critical of yourself, or feeling irritable and quick to anger. Doctors would also look to see whether there have been gains or losses in weight, changes in appetite, disturbances of sleep (difficulty in getting to sleep, or waking early), and feeling slowed down or agitated for much of the day.

The fact that doctors use this collection of features to diagnose depression has a vitally important message: **it means these feelings and changes are all *common symptoms of depression*—*not* signs of personal failing and inadequacy.**

If we can see negative states of mind for what they really are, we can take them less personally, we react with less aversion, and we have a chance to act in ways that will let the states of mind pass, rather than get us stuck even deeper in them.

How do you respond to these ideas? How might they be relevant to you? Do they seem to fit your own experience? You might like to make a note of your thoughts:

_____

_____

_____

_____

_____

_____

_____

Daily Practice

During Week 4, practice these exercises **for 6 out of the next 7 days**:

1. Sitting Meditation (or Sitting Meditation on Days 1, 3, and 5 and Mindful Walking or Mindful Movement on Days 2, 4, and 6)
2. 3-Minute Breathing Space—Regular
3. Additional Breathing Spaces (whenever needed)
4. Mindful Walking

1. Sitting Meditation: Mindfulness of Breath, Body, Sounds, and Choiceless Awareness

Each day this week, practice the guided sitting meditation on audio track 11 (*Sitting Meditation*); written instructions are given here:

SITTING MEDITATION: MINDFULNESS OF BREATH, BODY, SOUNDS, THOUGHTS, AND CHOICELESS AWARENESS

1. Practice mindfulness of breath and body, as described earlier (pages 88–89), until you feel reasonably settled.

2. Allow the focus of your awareness to shift from sensations in your body to **hearing**. Bring your attention to your ears and then allow the awareness to open and expand so that there is a receptiveness to sounds as they arise, wherever they arise.

3. There is no need to go searching for sounds or listening for particular sounds. Instead, as best you can, simply open your awareness so that it is receptive to sounds from all directions as they arise—sounds that are close, sounds that are far away, sounds that are in front, behind, to the side, above, or below. Open to a whole space of sound around you. Be aware of obvious sounds and of more subtle sounds, aware of the space between sounds, aware of silence.

4. As best you can, be aware of sounds simply as sensations. When you find that you are thinking *about* the sounds, reconnect, as best you can, with direct awareness of their sensory qualities (patterns of pitch, timbre, loudness, and duration), rather than their meanings or implications.

5. Whenever you notice that your awareness is no longer focused on sounds in the moment, gently acknowledge where your mind has moved and then retune your awareness back to sounds as they arise and pass from one moment to the next.

6. Mindfulness of sound can be a very valuable practice on its own, as a way of expanding awareness and giving it a more open, spacious quality, whether or

not the practice is preceded by awareness of body sensations or followed, as here, by awareness of thoughts.

7. When you are ready, let go of awareness of sounds and refocus your attention, so that your objects of awareness are now thoughts as events in the mind. Just as with sounds you focused awareness on whatever sounds arose, noticing them arise, develop, and pass away, so now, as best you can, bring awareness to thoughts that arise in your mind in just the same way—noticing when thoughts arise, focusing awareness on them as they pass through the space of your mind and eventually disappear. There is no need to try to make thoughts come or go. Just let them arise naturally, in the same way that you related to sounds arising and passing away.

8. Some people find it helpful to bring awareness to thoughts in the mind in the same way that they might if the thoughts were projected on the screen at the cinema. You sit, watching the screen, waiting for a thought or image to arise. When it does, you pay attention to it so long as it is there "on the screen," and then you let it go as it passes away. Alternatively, you might find it helpful to see thoughts as clouds or birds moving across a vast spacious sky or as leaves moving on a stream, carried by the current.

9. If any thoughts bring with them intense feelings or emotions, pleasant or unpleasant, as best you can, note their "emotional charge" and intensity and just let them be as they already are.

10. If at any time you feel that your mind has become unfocused and scattered, or it keeps getting repeatedly drawn into the drama of your thinking and imagining, you may like to notice where this is affecting your body. Often, when we don't like what is happening, we feel a sense of contraction or tightness in the face, shoulders, or torso and a sense of wanting to "push away" our thoughts and feelings. See if you notice any of this going on for you when some intense feelings arise. Then, once you have noticed this, see if it is possible to come back to the breath, and a sense of your body as a whole sitting and breathing, and use this focus to anchor and stabilize your awareness.

11. At a certain point you might like to explore the possibility of letting go of any particular object of attention, like the breath, sounds, or thoughts, and let the field of awareness be open to whatever arises in the landscape of your mind and your body and the world. This is sometimes called "choiceless awareness." See if it is possible to simply rest in awareness itself, effortlessly knowing whatever arises from moment to moment. That might include the breath, sensations from the body, sounds, thoughts, or feelings. As best you can, just sit, completely awake, not holding on to anything, not looking for anything, having no agenda whatsoever other than embodied wakefulness.

12. And when you are ready to bring the sitting to a close, perhaps return for a few minutes to the simple practice of mindful awareness of the breath.

Each time you begin this practice, remind yourself to **look out for experiences of aversion:**

- Move in close to any uncomfortable or unpleasant feelings, sensations, or thoughts and notice how you are reacting to them, **especially in the body.**
- See if you can, little by little, come to recognize the effects of aversion. What does aversion feel like? Where and how do you experience it in the body? What effect does it have on your thinking?
- What is your own "aversion signature" (the characteristic pattern of body sensations by which you recognize that aversion is present)?
- As you get to know aversion, see if it's helpful to actually say to yourself "Here's aversion" whenever you notice it arising.
- From day to day, make a note of your observations in the spaces provided.

Day 1: When you encountered unpleasant thoughts, feelings, or sensations, where were the sensations most intense in the body?

_____

_____

_____

_____

_____

What else did you notice during the sitting?

_____

_____

_____

_____

_____

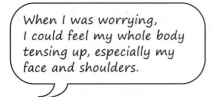

When I was worrying, I could feel my whole body tensing up, especially my face and shoulders.

Great noticing! Keep on exploring where the body reacts most intensely. It may be the same each time, or it may be different. The act of bringing gentle, interested, mindful awareness to investigate is itself healing.

Investigating experience here means bringing a kind, interested attention *to* the experience itself, rather than thinking analytically *about* the experience.

Investigation reveals and heals.

Day 2: What differences in awareness did you notice between when you focused on the breath and when you focused on sound?

_____

_____

_____

_____

_____

I also noticed:

_____

_____

_____

_____

I loved the sense of spaciousness and openness with sound!

Yes, it can feel like opening all the doors and windows of the mind! You are learning how to focus narrowly (the breath) and widely (sound/choiceless awareness). Both are very useful. So is knowing how and when to move from one to the other.

FOCUSED ATTENTION AND SPACIOUS ATTENTION

This week's meditation begins by FOCUSING attention on the breath. Then attention EXPANDS—to a more spacious sense of the whole body, then to sounds and the space around you, and finally to SPACIOUS choiceless awareness.

Both focused and spacious attention are invaluable in working with aversion:

Focused attention steadies and gathers the mind, helping you **stay present** in the face of unpleasant or uncomfortable experiences. It helps you **reconnect with the here and now** when the mind's automatic reactions are taking you away to the past, into the future, or urging you to tune out into a state of unawareness.

Spacious attention helps you be aware of the bigger picture—not just unpleasant experience, but also **how you are relating** to the experience. It allows you to see if there is aversion around.

Spacious attention gently counters the **contracting** effects of aversion on body and mind—creating a sense of **expansion and inclusion**.

It also allows a more **balanced view**. In aversion attention narrows to focus only on what is unpleasant—it can then seem that *all* experience is a problem. Widening the focus to also include other parts of the body, or other aspects of experience, allows what is problematic to be held together with what is okay—we can then see that not everything is a problem!

Day 3: What happens when you resist unpleasant feelings? Does it feel pleasant or unpleasant?

_____

_____

_____

_____

_____

I also noticed:

_____

_____

_____

_____

I'm puzzled. When I worry or ruminate about feeling sad, I'm focusing _on_ my emotions—but rumination, etc., are said to be forms of aversion, which is about wanting to _avoid_ experiencing unpleasant feelings. Can you clarify?

When we ruminate or worry, we are _thinking about_ painful emotions— _NOT_ actually _feeling_ them directly. Rumination and worry are subtle ways to avoid _experiencing the full intensity_ of unpleasant and painful feelings. And the thinking is all about finding ways to be rid of the unwanted emotions or reduce any threat.

Day 4: How did you respond to any sensations of physical discomfort?

_____

_____

_____

_____

_____

What else did you notice in this sitting?

_____

_____

_____

_____

I find that if I sit for a long time, my legs fall asleep and my back aches. I don't want to move, but sometimes it gets too painful not to.

You might like to try deliberately, and very gently, focusing your attention on the part of the body where the experience of discomfort is most intense, bringing awareness right into the sensations there. Continue to explore the sensations, knowing that it is fine to bring attention back to the breath, or to move mindfully, at any time.

PRACTICING WITH INTENSE SENSATIONS OF PHYSICAL DISCOMFORT

Physical discomfort provides a wonderful opportunity to learn how to relate more skillfully to **all** kinds of unwanted experience—including **emotional** discomfort. These skills will free you from getting trapped in depression, anxiety, and stress.

When you become aware of physical discomfort, see if it's possible to intentionally bring your attention **right into** the part of the body where the experience of discomfort is most intense. Once there, explore with **gentle**, interested attention the detailed pattern of sensations:

What, precisely, do the sensations feel like? Where exactly are they? Do they vary over time? Do they vary from one part of the region of intensity to another? The idea is not so much to think about the sensations as to sense and experience them directly. You can use the breath to carry awareness into such regions of intensity, "breathing into" them, just as in the body scan.

By deliberately moving your attention **toward** and **right into** the region of intensity, you reverse aversion's automatic tendency to **move away** from and **avoid unpleasant experiences.** You also give yourself the chance to see aversion, itself, more clearly. You may even begin to see the pains in the body for what they really are—not "big bad things" that we have to get rid of or away from at all costs, but constantly shifting and moving patterns of physical sensations that can be held in awareness and known.

Day 5: When you became aware of aversion, how did you respond to it?

_____

_____

_____

_____

Anything else that struck you as interesting?

_____

_____

_____

> I tried to stop the sense of "not wanting" and pushing away, but it didn't work—in fact, it just seemed to make things worse.

> You've noticed something really important. Once we see the problems aversion can create, it's natural to try to get rid of it—but that's just piling on more aversion. The best way to respond to aversion is to recognize it for what it is (perhaps saying "aversion" to yourself), treat it with respect, and let it be there until it passes in its own time, continuing to explore how it affects your body, with as gentle and soft awareness as possible.

The skillful response to aversion is to
(1) recognize it for what it is, (2) name it ("aversion"),
(3) treat it with respect, willingly allowing it to be present
until it passes, as (4) you continue to explore, with gentle
soft attention, how it affects your body.

Day 6: Look out for how aversion usually affects your body—perhaps frowning, tightness in your chest or stomach, tension in your shoulders. This is your "aversion signature"—write it in the box below.

My Aversion Signature Is:

_____

_____

What else did you notice?

_____

_____

_____

> It varies a bit from time to time, but most often I feel aversion as a contraction of the forehead, tension in the shoulders, and clenching my hands.

> Seeing all that is really helpful. You can now use that pattern of body sensations as a cue to tip you off that you are reacting with aversion—we'll say more about what you do then next week.

2. The 3-Minute Breathing Space—Regular

Every day this week, take a 3-minute breathing space three times a day, at the times you have chosen in advance, just as you did last week.

See if it's possible to guide yourself through all these breathing spaces without the help of the audio track. Of course, if you think it would be helpful to refresh your memory of the instructions, it's fine to use the audio or the instructions on page 98 when you need to.

Keep track of daily practice of these **R**EGULAR breathing spaces, circling an R here for every one you take at the end of the day (you can note them at the time on your smart phone or on a piece of notepaper):

Day 1: **R**   **R**   **R**   Day 2: **R**   **R**   **R**   Day 3: **R**   **R**   **R**

Day 4: **R**   **R**   **R**   Day 5: **R**   **R**   **R**   Day 6: **R**   **R**   **R**

3. Additional Breathing Spaces

Every day this week, in addition to your planned Regular Breathing Space, take additional breathing spaces *whenever in everyday life you notice unpleasant feelings, or a sense of tightening or holding in the body, or of being overwhelmed or knocked off balance.*

> ### Using Additional Breathing Spaces in Everyday Life
>
> In using breathing spaces in everyday life, you acknowledge that there is strong emotion around and take a few moments to bring awareness to it (as thoughts, feelings, and body sensations), simply allowing it to be there without judging it, without trying to chase it away or solve any problem (Step 1).
>
> You then "touch base," wherever you are, by returning to the anchor of the breath (Step 2) and to the grounded spaciousness of awareness of your body as a whole (Step 3). In this way you shift mental gears so that you bring a more responsive, balanced mind to the next moments of your day.
>
> Taking a breathing space will not necessarily mean that unpleasant feelings will no longer be present—the crucial thing is that your mind is now in a position to **respond** to them mindfully, rather than **react** to them automatically with aversion.

Whenever possible, do the full 3-minute practice. In situations where that isn't practical, see how creative you can be in adapting the breathing space to the situation—in a time of great busyness you might just momentarily bring awareness to what is going on in your mind and body, touch base with the breath, and then get a sense of your body as a whole.

The vital thing is to get into the habit of *responding* to unpleasant and difficult situations by intentionally stepping out of automatic pilot, rather than reacting automatically with aversion.

The breathing space will become the cornerstone of the MBCT program.

The cornerstone of the whole MBCT program is learning to respond to unpleasant and difficult experiences by, as a first step, intentionally taking a breathing space rather than reacting automatically with aversion.

Keep track of daily practice of these additional breathing spaces on a card you carry around or on your smart phone and then, at the end of the day, circle an X here for every time you take one:

Day 1: X X X X X   Day 2: X X X X X   Day 3: X X X X X

Day 4: X X X X X   Day 5: X X X X X   Day 6: X X X X X

For your records, you might like to describe here, in detail, one of your experiences in using an additional breathing space when a situation needed it:

> **Louis:** "Today I had a difficult phone call to make, and normally that would go round and round in my mind. I made the phone call, and I was able to deal with the call, but usually after a conversation like that, I would be worrying about it for ages. This time, afterwards, it was great. I stopped thinking about it. It didn't go on and on. Using the breathing space was amazing to me. It seemed to take the worry right away from me that would have been churning in my mind all afternoon."

The breathing space will offer you opportunity after opportunity to become acquainted with aversion in everyday life and to respond wisely to it.

How can we help ourselves remember the way aversion makes unpleasant experiences even worse?

Many people have found the following image, used for more than 2,500 years, a useful reminder.

The Two Arrows

If we were hit by an arrow, we would all experience physical pain and discomfort.

But for most of us it is as if, following this first arrow, we are then hit by a second arrow—aversion—the suffering arising from the reactions of anger, fear, grief, or distress that we add to the pain and discomfort from the first arrow.

More often than not, it is this second arrow that causes us the greater unhappiness. The crucial message of this image is that we can learn to free ourselves from the suffering of the second arrow.

Why? Because we fire it at ourselves!

---

4. Mindful Walking

Aversion is a powerful influence, taking you away from being fully present in each moment.

Establishing a mindful presence in your body from moment to moment—being fully here, now—is one of the most powerful ways to protect your mind from the dangers of aversion.

A calm, gathered, steady mind is simply less likely to get caught in the storms of aversion.

With your mind grounded in the body, your "feet firmly on the ground," you have something of the strength, stability, and dignity of a mountain that can endure all extremes of weather unmoved.

You probably spend some time each day walking, even if it's only from the parking lot or bus stop to your place of work or from one place to another at work or at home. These times provide precious opportunities to use the body to connect with mindful presence. You are walking anyway—can you do it mindfully?

You can kick-start your practice of mindful walking in everyday life with the formal practice of walking meditation. The instructions are on audio track 7 (*Mindful Walking*) and are summarized here:

MINDFUL WALKING

1. Find a place where you can walk up and down without feeling concerned about whether people can see you. It can be inside or outside—and the length of your walk may vary: perhaps between 5 and 10 paces.

2. Stand at one end of your walk, with your feet parallel to each other, about 4 to 6 inches apart, and your knees unlocked, so that they can flex gently. Allow your arms to hang loosely by your sides or hold your hands loosely together in front of your body. Direct your gaze, softly, straight ahead.

3. Bring the focus of your awareness to the bottoms of your feet, getting a direct sense of the physical sensations of the contact of your feet with the ground and the weight of your body transmitted through your legs and feet to the ground. You may find it helpful to flex your knees slightly a few times to get a clearer sense of the sensations in your feet and legs.

4. When you are ready, transfer the weight of your body into the right leg, noticing the changing pattern of physical sensations in your legs and feet as the left leg "empties" and the right leg takes over the support of the rest of the body.

5. With the left leg "empty," allow your left heel to rise slowly from the floor, noticing the sensations in the calf muscles as you do so, and continue, allowing the whole of the left foot to lift gently until only your toes are in contact with the floor. Aware of the physical sensations in the feet and legs, slowly lift the left foot, carefully move it forward, feeling the foot and leg as they move through the air, and place your heel on the floor. Allow the rest of the bottom of the left foot to make contact with the floor as you transfer the weight of the body into the left leg and foot, aware of the increasing physical sensations in the left leg and foot and of the "emptying" of the right leg and the right heel leaving the floor.

6. With the weight fully transferred to the left leg, allow the rest of your right foot to lift, and move it slowly forward, aware of the changing patterns of physical sensations in the foot and leg as you do so. Focusing your attention

on the right heel as it makes contact with the ground, transfer the weight of the body into the right foot as it is placed gently on the ground, aware of the shifting pattern of physical sensations in the two legs and feet.

7. In this way, slowly move from one end of your walk to the other, aware particularly of the sensations in the bottoms of your feet and heels as they make contact with the floor and of the sensations in the muscles of your legs as they swing forward.

8. At the end of your walk, stop for a few moments, then slowly turn around, aware of and appreciating the complex pattern of movements through which the body changes direction, and continue walking.

9. Walk up and down in this way, being aware, as best you can, of physical sensations in the feet and legs and of the contact of your feet with the floor. Keep your gaze directed softly ahead.

10. When you notice that your mind has wandered away from awareness of the sensations of walking, gently escort the focus of attention back to the sensations in your feet and legs, using the sensations as your feet contact the floor, in particular, as an "anchor" to reconnect with the present moment, just as you used the breath in the sitting meditation. If you find your mind has wandered, you might find it helpful to stand still for a few moments, gathering the focus of attention before resuming your walking.

11. Continue to walk for 10 to 15 minutes, or longer if you wish.

12. To begin with, walk at a pace that is slower than usual, to give yourself a better chance to be fully aware of the sensations of walking. Once you feel comfortable walking slowly with awareness, you can experiment as well with walking at faster speeds, up to and beyond normal walking speed. If you are feeling particularly agitated, it may be helpful to begin walking fast, with awareness, and to slow down naturally as you settle.

13. As often as you can, bring the same kind of awareness that you cultivate in walking meditation to your normal, everyday experiences of walking.

There's no need to do this formal practice every day this week (although you are very welcome to do so). Just practice it often enough to tune in to the simple power of staying mindfully present in your body as you walk.

You can then reconnect with the same sense of mindful presence as often as you remember, as you walk from one place to another in the course of your everyday life this week. Many people grow to love this practice.

Suzanne: *"I like walking meditation, because I can be conscious of it when I leave work. I have to pick up the kids, and sometimes I'm marching up the path to get to the school. I often find I am stomping and marching because I'm in a rush and getting a bit stressed.*

"Sometimes now I'll be aware of it, and I'll walk more slowly and, you know, breathe with the steps. So by the time I actually get to the kids waiting at the top of the path, I'm composed.

"If I slow down, everything else slows down and I become more aware of what's going on. And what might just take me ten seconds to get to the top of the path is then thirty or forty seconds, which is well worth it.

"It doesn't matter if I'm a few seconds late. When you become aware of time, I think one minute can be a very, very long time when you want it to be."

In mindful walking, you walk, knowing that you are walking, feeling the walking, being fully present with each step, walking for its own sake, without any destination. The focus is on maintaining moment-to-moment awareness of the sensations accompanying your movements, letting go of any thoughts or feelings about the sensations themselves.

We wish you well with your practice for Week 4.

Wild Geese

You do not have to be good.
You do not have to walk on your knees
for a hundred miles through the desert, repenting.
You only have to let the soft animal of your body
 love what it loves.
Tell me about despair, yours, and I will tell you mine.
Meanwhile the world goes on.
Meanwhile the sun and the clear pebbles of the rain
are moving across the landscapes,
over the prairies and the deep trees,
the mountains and the rivers.
Meanwhile the wild geese, high in the clear blue air,
are heading home again.
Whoever you are, no matter how lonely,
the world offers itself to your imagination,
calls to you like the wild geese, harsh and exciting—
over and over announcing your place
in the family of things.

MARY OLIVER

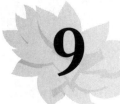

Week 5:
Allowing Things to Be
as They Already Are

Orientation

Unpleasant feelings are part and parcel of life. In themselves they may be quite challenging. Whether or not these feelings cause us further problems depends very much on how we respond to them.

If we react to unpleasant feelings with aversion, they'll most likely escalate—and we'll soon be stuck once more in unhappiness, stress, and depression.

The MBCT course invites us to explore another possibility—to discover that with awareness there is a different, more skillful way to respond to what is difficult and unpleasant in life—a way that really does offer a path to greater freedom.

WAITING IN LINE

Yoshi had finished his weekly shopping at the supermarket and surveyed the long checkout lines. He was usually pretty good at figuring out the fastest line to join. Today he got in a line that looked longer than some others but in which everyone had only a few items to buy. He smiled at his clever choice.

The first two customers checked out quickly, and now there were just two ahead of him. The first changed her mind about one of her purchases and asked the cashier for a replacement. He disappeared for a few minutes before returning with the right item. Yoshi could feel a mounting sense of irritation.

The next customer was eager to engage the cashier in a long discussion of last night's ball game. Yoshi could feel mounting frustration and anger.

At last they were done and it was Yoshi's turn. The cashier looked at him, smiled, and with a quick "Sorry, break time—someone else will be right here," disappeared. Yoshi felt a surge of helpless fury, and, as he waited, rehearsed with increasing rage the speech of protest and complaint he would make to the management.

And as he did so he became aware of a vague sense of tension and discomfort in his body, enough to remind him of an idea he'd recently encountered in his mindfulness classes—the aversion signature. He quickly scanned his body and found his torso knotted in tension, a painful intensity in the center of his chest. He took his awareness right into it, making direct contact with the fierce intensity of the body sensations and the sense of resistance to them, breathing into them, breathing out from them.

And, to Yoshi's amazement, the intensity, the anger, and the frustration fell away in a moment—just like that. Lost for words, Yoshi simply smiled at the new cashier as she took her place at the cash register and began packing his purchases.

When Yoshi deliberately turned **toward** painful emotions and aversion, as he experienced them **in the body**, they disappeared, almost miraculously.

How can we understand what happened here? It's not difficult to see that the situation triggered feelings of frustration. Aversion to these feelings then took over and locked Yoshi's mind/body into a feedback loop: frustration→anger→aversion→anger→aversion, and so on.

These loops rooted in aversion and **avoidance** were what was actually maintaining the anger. In his simple but fundamental gesture of **approach**—turning mindfully toward the feelings in his body—Yoshi, at a stroke, stopped feeding these self-perpetuating loops. The result was instant peace.

Such experiences powerfully reinforce the central message of MBCT: **it is *our relationship* to what is difficult and unpleasant that keeps us stuck in suffering—not the unpleasant feelings and sensations themselves.**

But changes as dramatic as Yoshi's don't always happen. More often, simply turning toward the difficult may weaken aversion, but it still leaves us experiencing some unpleasant feelings—to which we can then react with further aversion.

So, what do we do then?

This is where we learn to allow and let be.

Allowing and Letting Be

Allowing difficult feelings, thoughts, sensations, and inner experiences means that we willingly let them remain in awareness, without demanding that they change or be other than they are. Rather than getting into an argument with life, we allow our experience to be just as it already is.

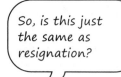

So, is this just the same as resignation?

Definitely not! In resignation we don't want to be having the experience we are having, but we feel helpless to do anything about it—all we can do is passively put up with it. Allowing/letting be involves an active, willing gesture of acceptance and openness to experience. It takes conscious commitment and energy. In allowing/letting be we _choose_ how to respond, rather than let ourselves be victims of the automatic habitual reaction of aversion.

Holding something gently in awareness is an affirmation that we can face it, name it, and work with it.

Allowing and letting be is not something most of us are used to. It's also not easy to get across the full flavor of this radical shift in our relationship with difficult experiences.

The poem "The Guest House" by the 13th-century poet Rumi communicates very powerfully the dramatic shift in attitude that is asked of us.

The Guest House

This being human is a guest house.
Every morning a new arrival.

A joy, a depression, a meanness,
some momentary awareness comes
as an unexpected visitor.

Welcome and entertain them all!
Even if they're a crowd of sorrows,
who violently sweep your house
empty of its furniture,

still, treat each guest honorably.
He may be clearing you out
for some new delight.

The dark thought, the shame, the malice,
meet them at the door laughing,
and invite them in.

Be grateful for whoever comes,
because each has been sent
as a guide from beyond.

RUMI

What strikes you most about this poem? Read it through and underline any words or lines that particularly catch your attention. Jot down your comments or reflections here:

_____

_____

_____

_____

_____

_____

_____

_____

_____

This is totally unrealistic! I just can't do this.

The poem makes its point by expressing the attitude of welcoming acceptance with dramatic intensity—but it really _is_ possible for any of us to begin to practice and cultivate a new relationship to difficult experiences. You can check this out for yourself, starting right now with the practices for this week.

How can I be expected to like depression, shame, or meanness?

It's really good to get this one clear. We don't actually have to _like_ unpleasant thoughts and feelings—just as an innkeeper wouldn't actually like every guest who arrives at his door. But equally, he wouldn't slam the door shut in their face! Treating all guests honorably, he would let them in, allow them to stay as long as they need to, and let them go when they are ready to leave. Can we treat the guests visiting our minds in the same way?

OK, how _do_ I treat the visitors to my mind honorably?

As best you can, you treat all experience with respect and care. You seek connection and engagement with it. You allow your experience, whatever it is, even the experience of aversion, to be held in awareness, just as it is, without requiring or demanding that it be different from what it is in this moment.

I have someone in my life right now who is causing lots of problems for me. . . . very abusive and unkind to me and the children. How can I be expected to allow this?

It's really important to understand that we're talking about allowing our own feelings, not allowing any treatment imposed on us by others. The first step in allowing is to see clearly what is actually happening. If there is something terribly wrong with a relationship, we may need to take action. Many of us put up with things for too long because we don't allow ourselves to see—really see—what is actually going on. We may have blamed ourselves for it all, or get trapped into thinking that we can change someone, when the person has no intention or capacity to change. Allowing your _feelings_ to be here, embracing them with kindness and compassion, may allow you to see the way forward more clearly.

Why Is It So Important to Cultivate Allowing/Letting Be?

Whenever we experience unpleasant feelings, sensations, or thoughts, we are at a choice point in our life's journey.

The choice we make will affect our happiness both immediately and farther down the road.

Choice 1: We react automatically with aversion—the need to get rid of the negative feelings, physical sensations, or thoughts.

With this reaction, the mind/body forges the first link in a chain of reactions that will get us stuck once more in unwanted, painful emotional states.

Choice 2: As best we can, we consciously embody the intention to allow the negative feelings, sensations, and thoughts to be here, even if we don't like them.

Taking this path, we take a significant and powerful step to incline the mind in a new direction—we shift our basic stance from one of "not wanting" to one of "opening."

This allows the chain of habitual automatic reactions to be broken at the first link. Experience then unfolds in new directions and we are less likely to get mired in the self-blame of depression, the terrors of anxiety, the red haze of anger, or the exhaustion of stress.

Holding unpleasant experiences in awareness without an immediate knee-jerk reaction of aversion dissolves, right there and then, the suffering caused by the struggle to get rid of them.

> Shifting our basic stance toward experience, from one of "not wanting" to one of "opening," allows the chain of habitual automatic reactions to be broken at the first link.

It also gives us a chance to explore for ourselves two of the "truths" of meditation traditions that are said to apply to every single difficult experience in life:

- **All unpleasant feelings pass of their own accord if we do not force them.**
- **There is a kind of peace and contentment we can experience even in the presence of unpleasant feelings.**

Daily Practice

During Week 5, practice each of these exercises **for 6 out of the next 7 days:**

1. Sitting Meditation: Working with Difficulties
2. 3-Minute Breathing Space—Regular
3. 3-Minute Breathing Space—Responsive, with added instructions

1. Sitting Meditation: Working with Difficulties

> To be at ease, we let go of the struggle of needing to make things different.

There are three steps to cultivating allowing and letting be in the face of difficult and unwanted experience:

Step 1

Deliberately and intentionally take your awareness to wherever in the body the sensations related to the unpleasant experience are most intense. Even if the most obvious features of the difficulty are negative thoughts or feelings, when you look carefully you will usually find somewhere in the body where there are sensations that have a felt connection to the experience.

Step 2

Bring a **gentle**, **kindly** awareness to how you are relating **in the body** to that experience—to any sense of contraction, pushing away, not wanting. Can you sense the reaction of aversion in the body?

Step 3

As best you can, **continue** to bring an **interested**, **friendly** awareness to the body sensations connected to the difficult experience **and the aversion** to it **as you allow them to be here**. As you hold sensations in awareness, **investigate** them with a gentle curiosity—staying connected to the experience as you let it be here.

   On Days 1, 3, and 5, practice the Working with Difficulty Meditation (audio track 12), summarized below.

   On Days 2, 4, and 6, practice sitting meditation as you did in Week 4 (pages 115–116) but without guidance from the audio, in silence, remembering to respond skillfully to any naturally arising difficulties as best you can.

**INVITING DIFFICULTY IN
AND WORKING WITH IT THROUGH THE BODY**

1. To begin, practice mindfulness of breath and body, as described earlier (pages 88–89), until you feel reasonably settled, then, when you are ready, follow this additional guidance as best you can.

2. Up till now, when you have been sitting and you have noticed that your mind has been pulled away to painful thoughts or emotions, the instructions

have been simply to notice where the mind has gone, then gently and firmly escort your attention back to the breath or body, or back to whatever you had intended to focus on.

3. Now you can explore a different way to respond. Instead of bringing attention back from a painful thought or feeling, now allow the thought or feeling to *remain* in the mind. Then, shifting your attention into the body, see if you can become aware of any physical sensations in the body that come along with the thought or emotion.

4. Then, when you have identified such sensations, deliberately move the focus of attention to the part of the body where these sensations are strongest. Perhaps imagining you could "**breathe into**" this region on the inbreath and "**breathe out**" from it on the outbreath, just as you practiced in the Body Scan—not to change the sensations but to explore them, to see them clearly.

5. If there are no difficulties or concerns coming up for you now and you want to explore this new approach, then, if you choose, you might *deliberately bring to mind a difficulty* that is going on in your life at the moment—something you don't mind staying with for a short while. It does not have to be very important or critical but something that you are aware of as somewhat unpleasant, something unresolved. Perhaps a misunderstanding or an argument, a situation where you feel somewhat angry, regretful, or guilty over something that has happened. If nothing comes to mind, you might choose something from the past, either recent or distant, that once caused unpleasantness.

6. Now, once you are focusing on some troubling thought or situation—some worry or intense feeling—allow yourself to take some time to tune in to any physical sensations in the body that the difficulty and your reaction to it evoke.

7. See if you are able to note, approach, and investigate inwardly what feelings are arising in your body, becoming mindful of those physical sensations, deliberately directing your focus of attention to the region of the body where the sensations are strongest in a gesture of an embrace, a welcoming.

8. This gesture might include breathing into that part of the body on the inbreath and breathing out from that region on the outbreath, exploring the sensations, watching their intensity shift up and down from one moment to the next.

9. Once your attention has settled on the bodily sensations and they are vividly present in the field of awareness, unpleasant as they may be, you might try deepening the attitude of acceptance and openness to whatever sensations you are experiencing by saying to yourself from time to time: *"It is here now. It is okay to be open to it. Whatever it is, it's already here. Let me be open to it."* Soften and open to the sensations you become aware of, intentionally letting go of tensing and bracing. Say to yourself: *"Softening," "Opening"* on each outbreath.

10. Then see if it is possible to stay with the awareness, exploring these bodily sensations and your relationship to them, breathing with them, accepting them, letting them be, allowing them to be just as they are.

11. Remember that, by saying *"It's already here"* or *"It's okay"* you are not judging the original situation or saying that everything's fine, but simply helping your awareness, right now, to remain open to the sensations in the body.

12. You do not have to *like* these feelings—it is natural not to want to have them around. You may find it helpful to say to yourself inwardly, *"It's okay not to want these feelings; they're already here; let me be open to them."*

13. If you choose, you can also experiment with holding in awareness both the sensations in the body and the feeling of the breath moving in and out, as you **breathe with** the sensations moment by moment.

14. And when you notice that the bodily sensations are no longer pulling your attention to the same degree, simply return 100% to sitting with the breath in the body as the primary object of attention.

15. If no powerful bodily sensations arise, feel free to try this exercise with any bodily sensations you notice, even if they have no emotional charge.

> Allowing experience means simply allowing space for whatever is going on, rather than trying to create some other state.

Every day, after your sitting meditation, jot down a few notes on your experience:

Day 1 (Audio):

Where in the body did you sense (1) any difficulty and (2) any aversion, not wanting, or resistance? What, if anything, happened to the difficulty and the aversion?

_____

_____

_____

_____

Anything else? _____

_____

_____

> I felt bad because I couldn't bring a difficulty to mind.

> No problem—this gives you a real "difficulty" in the moment to work with—the unpleasant feelings about not being able to do the practice as you would like to.

The difficulty you use for this practice can be something quite small—a slight sense of unease will do fine.

Day 2 (No audio):

Where in the body did you sense (1) any difficulty and (2) any aversion, not wanting, or resistance? What, if anything, happened to the difficulty and the aversion?

_____

_____

_____

_____

Anything else? _____

_____

_____

> It didn't work—the unpleasant feelings just didn't go away.

> That's perfectly okay. It's helpful to remember that, odd as it may seem, we're not actually trying to change the feelings themselves. The intention is to soften the way they are held in awareness—to ease our relationship of aversion to them—that's what makes us suffer and gets us stuck in emotional distress. Sometimes the feelings themselves change; often they don't.

Jayla: "When I brought the difficulty to mind, I felt it in my throat, just here. My throat felt tight, constricted, as if something was tied around my neck. It felt as if I might not be able to breathe—I didn't like it at all. I tried everything to deal with it—you know, breathing into it, relaxing, and all that. But it wouldn't go away. I started to panic a bit . . . what if it wouldn't go away? Then the voice on the CD said something about noticing how I was relating to the sensations in the body. I had not understood what this meant before; then I realized that it was referring not only to the feelings in my throat but also to the fact that <u>I did not want to have these feelings</u>!!! I thought to myself, 'Is there something I am not seeing here? Something I'm not feeling?' So I scanned my body again. I discovered that this 'not wanting' had its own set of physical sensations. They were not in my throat but in my abdomen. I started to bring my attention, very gently, to this region, and as soon as I did so, the feelings in my abdomen and my throat dissolved. I had not expected it. I think it helped that I was not trying to change things at this point. It was so clear I was really surprised and moved."

Like Jayla, with practice, you may sometimes be able to sense very clearly *in the body* the difference between the difficulty and the aversion to it—and to see that, even if you can do nothing about the difficulty itself, you can soften the aversion to it.

Day 3 (Audio):

Where in the body did you sense (1) any difficulty and (2) any aversion, not wanting, or resistance? What, if anything, happened to the difficulty and the aversion?

_____

_____

_____

_____

Anything else? _____

_____

_____

Day 4 (No audio):

Where in the body did you sense (1) any difficulty and (2) any aversion, not wanting, or resistance? What, if anything, happened to the difficulty and the aversion?

_____

_____

_____

_____

Anything else? _____

_____

_____

> A very old and familiar difficulty came up—I felt so angry with it for all the suffering it has caused—and with myself for not sorting it out before.

> At such times, you might find it helpful to remind yourself that kindness is the foundation of MBCT. Kindness to yourself means being gentle, perhaps saying to yourself, "It's okay not to like these feelings—it's okay not to want them around." Kindness to what's arising, moment by moment, is saying, "OK, you're here. Let me allow you to be here, even though I don't like you." We move in close. We open the guest house to what we fear; we roll out the red carpet.

We disempower aversion by intentionally bringing
to all experience a basic sense of _kindness_—
allowing the experience to be, just as it is,
without judging it or trying to make it different.

From this clear seeing we can choose what, if anything,
needs to change.

Day 5 (Audio):

Where in the body did you sense (1) any difficulty and (2) any aversion, not wanting, or resistance? What, if anything, happened to the difficulty and the aversion?

_____

_____

_____

_____

Anything else? _____

_____

_____

> I was thinking about my friend who has cancer. How can I say "It's okay" to that—because it isn't okay!

> Saying "It's okay" is not about the fact that your friend has cancer. The words are simply meant to help you, in that particular moment, to be with your feelings about that situation as they already are—the fear, anger, or guilt—with less struggle and aversion. You are gently encouraging yourself to feel what is already present, instead of fighting it—that's what "okay" means here.

Maria: "When I brought the difficulty to mind, a whole part of my body became really tight and knotted. And then I breathed into it, and it suddenly became like a great big empty space . . . with the air coming in and out. You know, when you come back from vacation, and you open all the doors and windows to let the air blow through . . . well, it was like that. . . . And the tension about the difficulty was still there. But I thought, 'Oh, you're still there, but never mind, the wind's blowing through, and that's all right.' There was more space for it, and I could sort of look at it.

"The feeling in my body was still a bit tight, but it was much smaller, and all the air was sort of flowing around it. At the beginning, it was the whole thing. Because I was so tight, you know, there was nothing else there. It was like a solid mass of rock. It was huge. It was so solid that you couldn't get around it, but then it shrank to a small stone. It was still stone . . . but it was small.

"It's really good. Because I think, probably, I have been pushing the issue away and sort of sitting on it and not letting it come up fully to the surface. I haven't allowed it before to simply be there. I thought it would just overwhelm me. Now I've found I can just be with it."

Allowing/letting be frees us from the contraction of
aversion. It creates a space where the difficult can be held
more kindly, with less struggle.

Very often, letting be will not immediately remove
the original unpleasant feeling.

Day 6 (No audio):
Where in the body did you sense (1) any difficulty and (2) any aversion, not
wanting, or resistance? What, if anything, happened to the difficulty and the
aversion?

_____

_____

_____

_____

Anything else? _____

_____

_____

2. 3-Minute Breathing Space—Regular

Every day this week, take a 3-minute breathing space three times a day, at the times you have decided in advance, just like you did last week. See if it's possible to do these without any help from the audio.

To keep track of your practice, at the end of each day, circle an **R** in the table below (Practice 3) for each of these planned breathing spaces you take.

3. 3-Minute Breathing Space—Responsive, with Added Instructions

Every day this week, in addition to the planned Regular Breathing Space, take a breathing space *whenever you notice any unpleasant feelings, tension, resistance, or sense of not wanting things to be as they are.*

You can keep the intention to do this practice alive by noting (on your smart phone or on a card you carry with you) each time you take a responsive breathing space, even if it's only very brief. At the end of each day, circle an **X** in the table for each breathing space taken.

DAY	REGULAR breathing space	RESPONSIVE breathing space									
DAY 1	R R R	X	X	X	X	X	X	X	X	X	X
DAY 2	R R R	X	X	X	X	X	X	X	X	X	X
DAY 3	R R R	X	X	X	X	X	X	X	X	X	X
DAY 4	R R R	X	X	X	X	X	X	X	X	X	X
DAY 5	R R R	X	X	X	X	X	X	X	X	X	X
DAY 6	R R R	X	X	X	X	X	X	X	X	X	X
DAY 7	R R R	X	X	X	X	X	X	X	X	X	X

You might like to explore using the extended instructions below (audio track 9, *3-Minute Breathing Space—Extended Version*):

USING THE BREATHING SPACE: EXTENDED INSTRUCTIONS

You have been practicing the breathing space regularly three times a day and whenever you need it. We have also suggested that whenever you feel troubled in body or mind, the first step is always to take a breathing space. Here is some extra guidance that may help at these times.

1. Awareness

You have already practiced bringing the focus of awareness to your inner experience and noticing what is happening in your thoughts, feelings, and bodily sensations.

Now you may find it helpful also to describe and identify what is arising—to put experiences into words (such as saying in your mind, "A feeling of anger is arising" or . . . "Self-critical thoughts are here").

2. Redirecting Attention

You have already practiced gently redirecting your full attention to the breath, following the breath all the way in and all the way out.

In addition, you might like to explore noting at the back of your mind: "Breathing in . . . Breathing out" or counting breaths from 1 to 5 and then starting over again: "Inhaling, 1 . . . exhaling, 1; Inhaling, 2 . . . ," and so forth.

3. Expanding Attention

You have already practiced allowing the attention to expand to the whole body, becoming aware of your posture and facial expression, holding in awareness all the sensations in your body right now, just as they are.

Now, if you choose, you can extend this step, especially if there is any sense of discomfort, tension, or resistance. If these sensations are present, you might bring your awareness to them by "breathing into" them on the inbreath and "breathing out" from the sensations, softening and opening with the outbreath, saying to yourself on the outbreath "It's okay . . . whatever it is, it's already here: let me feel it."

As best you can, bring this expanded awareness to the next moments of your day.

It seems odd to say "A feeling of anger is arising." Why not just say "I'm angry"?

Saying "The emotion of X is here" is simply describing your experience in the moment. Saying "I am X" reinforces the habit of identifying personally with the emotion—"It's me"—which is the beginning of all the stories we tell ourselves that get us stuck in rumination and worry. Changing how we talk to ourselves is a simple way to begin to take things less personally.

Isn't the responsive breathing space just another, clever way to fix things?

There's a fine line between using the breathing space as a way to allow your experience to be just as it is in the moment and using it in the hope that it will "work" to get rid of unpleasant feelings. The crucial thing is intention—whatever you do with the hidden agenda to get rid of unwanted feelings can easily backfire. The challenge is to be honest with yourself and, as best you can, explore the possibility of really "letting be" as an act of kindness.

Sometime this week, jot down a few notes here describing *one* occasion on which you found a responsive 3-minute breathing space helpful.

What was the difficulty? What was your response? What was the effect?

_____

_____

_____

_____

Chao: "I was going to visit my father in the hospital last Monday. You never know what you are going to find when you get there . . . you get so many mixed messages. So early Sunday morning, I woke up feeling really apprehensive and panicky. So I thought, 'Unpleasant event, unpleasant event, unpleasant event,' which I haven't actually done before. I thought, 'Now, what are you really feeling?'

"I was really pleased, because I was thinking, 'My tummy's churning, my hands are clenched. I'm having difficulty with breathing.'

". . . and then I started breathing . . . and it didn't progress . . . it didn't progress. I was really pleased because what it does is make you feel that everything isn't out of control. After all, it doesn't solve everything right away—those things were still there—but it did help. It did help."

The focus of this chapter has been on how you can cultivate a relationship of allowing/letting be to unwanted **emotional** pain. As we close, you might be interested to take a look at Lexy's description of how MBCT changed her relationship to **physical** pain:

Lexy: "In 2007 I had an accident that resulted in a severe back injury. This left me so debilitated and in so much pain I had to take a year off from college to recover.

"I eventually went back to my studies but had to continue to take high doses of medication to manage the pain.

"This spring I enrolled in the 8-week mindfulness course, which has transformed my life.

"It helped me develop awareness of my whole body, and through this awareness I was better able to cope with the pain. It taught me not to ignore the pain, but to accept its presence, which made it have less of an impact on my thoughts, feelings, and actions. I began to have a different relationship to my pain, to view it in a new way. It also helped me improve my posture.

"At the end of the course I have, for the first time, felt able to come off my pain medication and instead replaced it with the simple meditation practices/techniques I've learned, which are easily adaptable to everyday life."

Prelude

What if there is no need to change, no need to try to transform yourself into someone who is more compassionate, more present, more loving or wise?

How would this affect all the places in your life where you are endlessly trying to be better?

What if the task is simply to unfold, to become who you already are in your essential nature—gentle, compassionate, and capable of living fully and passionately present? . . .

What if the question is not why am I so infrequently the person I really want to be, but why do I so infrequently want to be the person I really am?

How would this change what you think you have to learn?

What if becoming who and what we truly are happens not through striving and trying but by recognizing and receiving the people and places and practices that offer us the warmth of encouragement we need to unfold?

How would this shape the choices you make about how to spend today?

What if you knew that the impulse to move in a way that creates beauty in the world will arise from deep within and guide you every time you simply pay attention and wait?

How would this shape your stillness, your movement, your willingness to follow this impulse, to just let go and dance?

ORIAH MOUNTAIN DREAMER

10

Week 6:
Seeing Thoughts *as* Thoughts

Orientation

John was on his way to school.

He was worried about the math lesson.

He was not sure he could control the class again today.

It was not part of a janitor's duty.

Before reading on, take a moment to jot down a few words describing how you understood these sentences as you read them:

_____

_____

_____

_____

_____

_____

Lou: *"First, I thought it was a little boy going to school, worried about a math lesson that was coming up. Then, suddenly, I realized it wasn't a boy at all, but a teacher. And then, with the last line, I had to do another mental switch to realize that it wasn't a teacher but the school janitor."*

This little exercise illustrates some very important points:

- Our minds are constantly "making meaning" out of what comes to us through our senses.

- Those meanings are often based on only a few, partial scraps of information—the meanings we make almost always go well beyond the bare facts given.

- As a result, the meanings we create often don't reflect a true picture of what's happening—that's why, as in the exercise, we have to update our views repeatedly in light of new information.

- Although we're constantly adding extra to the information we receive, unless someone comes along and plays a trick on us (as in the opening of this chapter), we're not aware that it is *we* who are actively making meaning—we think we are just seeing it as it is.

THE OFFICE

Take a few moments to imagine this scene as clearly as you can:

You are feeling down because you've just had a quarrel with a colleague at work. Shortly afterward, you see another colleague in the hall and he or she rushes off quickly, saying he or she can't stop.

Write down here the thoughts that would go through your mind:

_____

_____

_____

_____

_____

_____

_____

Now imagine this scene:

> *You are feeling happy because you and a work colleague have just been praised for good work. Shortly afterward, you see another colleague in the hall and he or she rushes off quickly, saying he or she can't stop.*

Write down the thoughts that would go through your mind:

_____

_____

_____

_____

_____

_____

Now look back over what you have written in response to the two scenarios.
    Make a note of anything that strikes you about your thoughts in the two situations:

_____

_____

_____

_____

_____

_____

_____

_____

_____

_____

Lou: "With the first scenario, I would think the colleague had dashed off because she was feeling hostile toward me or had heard something bad about me. It would keep going over and over in my mind: Why didn't she speak to me?

"In the second scenario, I would just think she had a meeting to go to. It would briefly occur to me she might be envious, but I wouldn't give it much thought."

Isn't that interesting? We have exactly the same objective situation—the colleague said she couldn't stop—but two very different interpretations, leading to very different feelings: upset and worry in one case, not bothered in the other.

The "extra" that our minds add will be different depending on the <u>frame of mind</u> we bring to our experience. Our frame of mind will reflect, among other things, what has just happened to us. The different interpretations reflect different <u>frames of mind</u>. The quarrel set up a self-critical frame of mind; the praise set up a more positive frame.

Frame of mind → Interpretation → Feelings

Our interpretations of events reflect what we bring to them as much as, or more than, what is actually there:

Thoughts are not facts
(Even the ones that say they are!)

Moods and feelings are powerful influences shaping our frame of mind—the lens through which we see the world. This, in turn, shapes our patterns of thinking.

In moods, thinking patterns often echo themes similar to the feelings that shaped them—hopeless feelings lead to hopeless thoughts, kind feelings lead to benevolent thoughts, and so on.

Feelings give birth to related thinking patterns.

When the themes of feelings and thoughts mesh in this way, those thinking patterns re-create the feelings that shaped them in the first place. As well as keeping the feelings going, the close link between feelings and thoughts makes the thoughts seem very real.

When thoughts and mood mesh, thoughts can be very compelling and hard to see *as* thoughts.

This is how the vicious cycles that keep us stuck in painful emotions keep going.

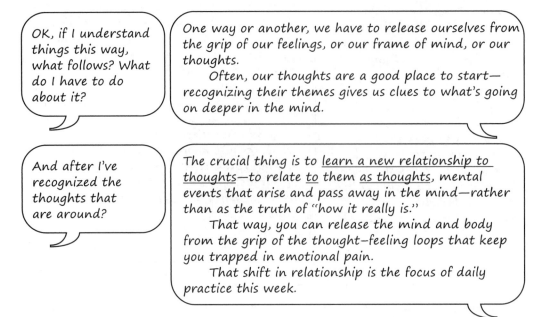

OK, if I understand things this way, what follows? What do I have to do about it?

One way or another, we have to release ourselves from the grip of our feelings, or our frame of mind, or our thoughts.
   Often, our thoughts are a good place to start—recognizing their themes gives us clues to what's going on deeper in the mind.

And after I've recognized the thoughts that are around?

The crucial thing is to <u>learn a new relationship to thoughts</u>—to relate <u>to</u> them <u>as thoughts</u>, mental events that arise and pass away in the mind—rather than as the truth of "how it really is."
   That way, you can release the mind and body from the grip of the thought–feeling loops that keep you trapped in emotional pain.
   That shift in relationship is the focus of daily practice this week.

Daily Practice

During Week 6, practice each of these exercises **for 6 out of the next 7 days**:

1. Sitting Meditation—with a focus on Relating to Thoughts as Mental Events

2. 3-Minute Breathing Space—Regular

3. 3-Minute Breathing Space—Responsive, with a Focus on Thoughts

In addition:

4. Setting up an Early Warning System

1. Sitting Meditation—with a Focus on Relating to Thoughts as Mental Events

Every day, practice guided sitting meditation for at least 40–45 minutes a day (choose from these audio tracks: *10-Minute Sitting Meditation, 20-Minute Sitting Meditation, Stretch and Breath Meditation, Sitting Meditation, Working with Difficulty Meditation*). You might make up the 40–45 minutes by combining two 20-minute meditations or one 20-minute plus two 10-minute meditations or just use one 40-minute meditation. Feel free to experiment with different combinations from day to day.

   Whatever meditations you use, remember to hold in mind the possibility of relating to thoughts *as* thoughts—passing mental events, not "you" or "the truth."

THREE WAYS TO PRACTICE
VIEWING THOUGHTS AS MENTAL EVENTS

Option 1: When you become aware that your attention has drifted away from your intended focus (breath, body, or sound, etc.), **pause** long enough to recognize any thoughts, images, or memories that are around. Then **say "thinking" to yourself**, very quietly, as a reminder to see these thoughts *as* thoughts, and, as gently and kindly as you can, return the attention to your intended focus of breath, body, sound, etc.

Option 2: Make thoughts themselves the primary focus of your attention. Just as, with *sounds*, you focus awareness on whatever sounds arise, noticing them arise, develop, and pass away, so now, as best you can, you bring awareness to *thoughts* that arise in your mind in just the same way.

Images or metaphors can help. You might bring awareness to thoughts:

- as if they were projected on the screen at the movie theater. You sit, watching the screen, waiting for a thought or image to arise. When it does, you pay attention to it so long as it is there "on the screen," and then you let it go as it passes away.
- as if they come onto an empty stage and exit through the opposite wing.
- as if the mind is a vast spacious sky and thoughts are clouds or birds passing through the sky.
- as if thoughts are leaves moving on a stream, carried by the current.

To begin with, aim to practice with thoughts as the main object of attention for no more than 3 or 4 minutes at a time—no one finds it easy to attend directly to thoughts in this way. Feel free to explore other images or metaphors or none at all.

Option 3: When you notice that thoughts have a strong emotional charge, or that they seem to be intrusive or persistent, you might remember that emotions are "packages" of body sensations, feelings, and related thoughts (pages 78, 151). Briefly acknowledge the thoughts *as* thoughts. Then **"drop down" below the thoughts to explore, in the body, the felt sense of the emotion that "gave birth" to the thoughts**. Bring awareness right up to and into the region of the body where these sensations are most intense—just as you did in working with difficulties last week.

Day 1:

What was the effect of reminding yourself to recognize thoughts as thoughts by pausing and saying "thinking" to yourself before returning to the breath?

_____

_____

_____

_____

What else did you notice?

_____

_____

_____

> I realized that "coming back to the breath" had become a bit automatic. It felt good to pause and take the time to see things more clearly and let go of thinking more consciously.

> That's good—the simple (but often not easy) movement of pausing, recognizing, labeling, and letting go of thoughts, repeated over and over again, is a very powerful way to build a different relationship to thoughts.

The Train of Associations

We do not need to fight with thoughts or struggle against them or judge them. Rather, we can simply choose not to follow the thoughts once we are aware that they have arisen.

When we lose ourselves in thought, identification is strong. Thought sweeps the mind and carries it away, and, in a very short time, we can be carried far indeed. We hop on a train of association, not knowing that we have done so, and certainly not knowing the destination. Somewhere down the line, we may wake up and realize that we have been thinking, that we have been taken for a ride. And when we step down from the train, it may be in a very different mental environment from where we jumped aboard.

As an exercise, you might close your eyes and imagine yourself sitting in a movie theater, watching an empty screen. Simply wait for thoughts to arise. What exactly are they? What happens to them? Thoughts are like magic displays, which seem real when we are lost in them but then vanish upon inspection.

But what about the strong thoughts that affect us? We are watching, watching, watching, and then, all of a sudden—whoosh! We are gone, lost in a thought. What is that about? What are the mind states or the particular kinds of thoughts that catch us again and again, so that we forget that they are just empty phenomena passing by?

The kinds of thoughts we have, and their impact on our lives, depend on our understanding of things. If we are in the clear, powerful space of just seeing thoughts arise and pass, then it does not really matter what kind of thinking appears in the mind; we can see our thoughts as the passing show that they are.

From thoughts come actions. From actions come all sorts of consequences. In which thoughts will we invest? Our great task is to see them clearly, so that we can choose which ones to act on and which simply to let be.

JOSEPH GOLDSTEIN

Day 2:

What happened when you made thoughts themselves the focus of your attention? Were any of the images or metaphors helpful?

_____

_____

_____

_____

Anything else?

_____

_____

_____

When I first tried to focus on thoughts, they disappeared completely! Then, when I focused on them like a movie, I could only remain "in the audience" for a few thoughts before I got drawn into the action. When I came to, I began thinking, I'll never be able to do this.

These are all very common experiences. It can be really helpful to include thoughts <u>about</u> the practice (such as "I'll never be able to do this") <u>in</u> the practice—to see <u>them</u> as passing mental events too. That way they won't upset or discourage you so much. You might play with relating to them as voices from the seat behind you in the theater.

That reminds me of something that happened one day last week. I was really struggling to concentrate on my meditation. My mind was all over the place with stuff that's going on at work. I kept saying to myself: Come back to the breath, come back to the breath, <u>come back to the breath</u>! I really thought it wasn't doing me any good—maybe actually making me worse. Then something happened. I realized "This is not doing me any good" was another thought—an insidious, hidden thought—and so was "It's making me worse." I'd been looking for thoughts on the stage, but these didn't appear on the stage at all. They came from somewhere else entirely, just as you said. But once I'd seen them, it was amazing—the feeling of hopelessness dissolved. The stuff about work was still around, but it didn't have the same sense of heaviness that it had had before. I ended up really curious as to how I can work on seeing this earlier, so I don't get taken in so easily.

Absolutely . . . it's as if some of these thoughts come in disguise, so you don't even see them creeping into your consciousness—they're too well camouflaged against the background of feelings, and then they get caught up in the reaction of "not wanting to have" these feelings. It can be so difficult, can't it? It can be really helpful to take a moment, listen for the "voice from behind you," and shift attention into the body to discover what emotions might be giving birth to these subtle thoughts.

Day 3:

How did you respond to any charged, intrusive, or persistent thoughts you encountered? What happened?

_____

_____

_____

_____

Anything else?

_____

_____

_____

> Worries about a meeting with my boss tomorrow kept forcing their way into my mind. I kept labeling them "thinking" and coming back to the breath, but they still just kept on coming up.

> Well done for persisting in that way. You might find it helpful to remember that emotionally charged thoughts are just the visible tip of the iceberg of most emotional "packages." The bulk of the 'berg—the body sensations and feelings—are submerged. Many people find this general rule helpful: <u>When emotion-related thoughts are around, acknowledge the thoughts, then drop down into the body to bring awareness to the sensations and feelings that gave birth to the thoughts.</u>

Mindfulness invites us to see thoughts as part
of a whole package. We focus directly on the _feeling_
that gives birth to the thought, rather than getting tangled
in thoughts themselves. Mindfully, gently we investigate:
"What am I feeling in this moment?"

Louise: "I had been having some difficult weeks and felt very low. I knew that, normally, there was every chance I would spiral down to a full depression. I was in the doctor's office with one of the children, feeling pressured because I'd had to take time off work to be there. Half of me was thinking, 'What will the boss say?' and the other half 'Why shouldn't I be here? I'm entitled to it,' and so on and so on.

"I noticed what was happening, but not in the old way, when I would tell myself not to be so stupid. Instead, I took a moment. I acknowledged what I was feeling: angry, tired, confused, and very worried about my daughter. Then I felt my perspective broaden, and I could say to myself, 'It's OK to feel like this; it's OK.' I allowed the feelings just to be there, without struggling to chase them away—and they just eased away."

Day 4:

What was your attitude toward the thoughts you encountered? Were you impatient, irritated, wishing they weren't there, or accepting, interested, or just neutral toward them?

_____

_____

_____

_____

Anything else?

_____

_____

_____

I surprised myself. Streams of worries and self-critical thoughts were cascading through my mind, as usual. But a corner of my mind remembered I could look <u>at</u> the thoughts. Then I became <u>interested</u> in them rather than swept away in the struggle with them.

Wonderful! That's the crucial shift in perspective the practice asks of us— mindfulness gives us another place to stand. When thoughts and feelings seem like a huge torrent, and it feels like we're being hurled down with the force of the water, we move to stand behind the waterfall. We watch the thoughts and feelings cascade past. They are very close. You feel the force of them, but they are not you.

As always, kindness is the foundation of skillful practice.

Kindness to your thoughts means gently reminding yourself
that thoughts are not the enemy—allowing them to be here,
holding them in a friendly, interested awareness.

Kindness to yourself means allowing yourself to be just
as you already are in this moment.

Day 5:

Make a note of any familiar, well-worn patterns of thinking you recognized. What effect did they have?

_____

_____

_____

_____

Anything else?

_____

_____

_____

So many old routines: I'm not good enough. I can't do this. What will happen if . . . ? All the usual suspects!

Humor is a great ally here. Once you can see these old patterns for what they really are, give them a wry smile, and welcome them in, however slightly. In this way, you begin to strip them of their power to upset and control you.

YOUR MIND'S TOP 10 UNHELPFUL THOUGHTS

When you've watched your mind a great deal and seen the same old thoughts come up again and again, you will eventually find you don't rise to the bait anymore.

Naming your familiar thought patterns can help you recognize them when they start up. It allows you to say, "Ah, I know this program. This is my 'I can't stand my boss' program or my 'No one recognizes how hard I work' program." The recognition of thought patterns for what they are creates space between you and them. Eventually you may see these familiar patterns so clearly that they will no longer press your buttons.

See if you can identify your own Top 10 unhelpful thought patterns or programs. Keep a record of these "usual suspects" here:

Program 1 _____

Program 2 _____

Program 3 _____

Program 4 _____

Program 5 _____

Program 6 _____

Program 7 _____

Program 8 _____

Program 9 _____

Program 10 _____

It's fine to make this a continuing project extending over the next few weeks—and you don't have to find 10! (Feel free to make extra copies or download this from *www.guilford.com/teasdale-materials*.)

Day 6:

What form do your thoughts take? Do you experience them as words, images or pictures, or wordless, imageless "meanings"? If words, what is the tone of voice?

Anything else?

> I seemed to experience a mixture. Some thoughts came clearly as words in my head—often in a nagging voice. Other times there were images: When I felt rejected I saw an image of friends huddled together laughing and talking among themselves, without me.

> Some people think mainly in words, others mainly in pictures. Sometimes there's just a sense of meaning without words or images. When the same emotions keep coming back, it's always worth checking for any images that seem to crystallize the essence of the feeling—they might just be keeping the emotion going.

"It is amazing to observe how much power we give unknowingly to uninvited thoughts: 'Do this, say that, remember, plan, obsess, judge.' They have the potential to drive us quite crazy, and they often do!" —Joseph Goldstein

2. The 3-Minute Breathing Space—Regular

Every day this week, take a 3-minute breathing space three times a day, at the times you have decided in advance, just like you did last week.

To keep track of your practice, at the end of each day, circle an **R** in the table on page 161 for each of these planned breathing spaces you took.

3. The 3-Minute Breathing Space—Responsive with a Focus on Thoughts

Every day this week, in addition to the planned Regular Breathing Space, take a breathing space *whenever you notice any unpleasant feelings and whenever you notice your thoughts are getting the better of you.*

You can help keep the intention for this practice alive by circling an **X** in the table below for each time you've used a responsive breathing space.

Day	REGULAR breathing space	RESPONSIVE breathing space
Day 1	R R R	X X X X X X X X X X
Day 2	R R R	X X X X X X X X X X
Day 3	R R R	X X X X X X X X X X
Day 4	R R R	X X X X X X X X X X
Day 5	R R R	X X X X X X X X X X
Day 6	R R R	X X X X X X X X X X
Day 7	R R R	X X X X X X X X X X

When thoughts threaten to overwhelm, taking a breathing space (no matter how briefly) is always the first step.

If negative thoughts are still around after you take a breathing space, you have a number of options for what to do next.

Option 1. You might just *re-enter* the flow of everyday life, with your perspective on thinking shifted, even if only slightly, by taking a breathing space.

Option 2. You might continue to be mindful of the emotion fueling the thoughts, focusing on how it is experienced in the *body*. You may find it useful to follow the extended instructions for Step 3 introduced last week (pages 144–145).

Option 3. You might focus on the negative *thoughts* themselves, exploring one or more of the strategies described in the box on page 162.

THE BREATHING SPACE: WAYS TO SEE THOUGHTS DIFFERENTLY

1. Simply watch the thoughts come and go in the field of awareness, without feeling you have to follow them.

2. Remind yourself to view the negative thoughts as mental events, rather than facts.

3. Write your thoughts down on paper. This helps you see them in a way that is less emotional and overwhelming. The pause between having the thought and writing it down provides an opportunity to take a wider perspective.

4. See if you recognize the thinking pattern as one of your "top ten" unhelpful thoughts.

5. Focus, with kindness and compassion, on the feelings that may be giving birth to the thoughts, asking yourself "What feelings are here now?" "How am I experiencing these feelings **in the body**?"

I'm getting a bit confused by all these different kinds of breathing spaces. How can I remember what they all are, and how do I know which one to use at a particular time?

In all difficult situations, the first step is always to take a basic breathing space. You can think of that step as taking you into a hall, out of which there are a number of doors—you leave the hall through one of them. Each door offers a different possibility for your next step: re-entry, body, and thoughts (next week we'll introduce one more door).

We encourage you to explore all the doors over time. That way you discover for yourself the most skillful response to each different kind of situation. As a general rule, it's usually helpful, at some point, to focus on the actual physical sensations in the body. Over time, you'll discover your own ways to use the breathing space so it becomes for you a faithful friend.

Sometime this week, jot down a few notes here describing **ONE** occasion on which you found a responsive breathing space to difficult thoughts helpful.

What were the thoughts? What was your response? What was the effect?

_____

_____

_____

_____

_____

_____

_____

> **Chan:** *"I'll suddenly think of something that somebody said 2 weeks ago—I bet she meant such and such. Why did she say that?—and my mind just races and races.*
>
> *"But then I think of that saying: Thoughts aren't facts. That one really clicked with me. Thoughts are not facts, and the other bit that said, even the ones that tell you they are, because if you've got that sort of thing going around in your head you can say, Now come on. That is not real. This is real. You're here in this room, and look at all the good things that are around you. And then the other thought would come back in: But she really did say that. That really did happen. And then I was able to pick up on the next phrase, even the ones that say they are [laughs]. Then I do the breathing space, and I usually find that it's gone."*

4. Setting Up an Early Warning System

The MBCT program was originally designed to develop the skills and understanding to empower people who had been depressed to take action to avoid getting deeply mired in depression again. The following section is written primarily with such people in mind.

However, we've also found that many people find it helpful to recognize the earliest signs that tell them they're getting burned out, overstressed, or overanxious. So, even if depression is not your main problem, you may find this section helpful.

Your actions will be most effective if you can respond
as early as possible to signs that your mood is worsening.

So, the first step in preparing an Early Warning System is to identify your **Early Warning Signs** (sometimes also called your **Relapse Signature**)—the pattern of signs that tell you that your mood is beginning to spiral down in ways that, if left unchecked, will get you stuck, once more, in depression or some other painful emotion.

Here are some of the signals of sinking mood that previous participants in MBCT have identified. Some may be true for you; others may not. You might like to check the box of any that seem to reflect your own experience:

Sleeping more or sleeping less, waking at different times, having difficulty getting to sleep ☐

Giving up on exercise ☐

Not wanting to see people ☐

Getting easily exhausted ☐

Not wanting to deal with business (opening mail, paying bills, etc.) ☐

Eating more or eating less, not interested in food ☐

Becoming irritable with yourself and other people ☐

Seeing negative thoughts and feelings take hold—finding them "sticky," difficult to dismiss ☐

Putting things off, postponing deadlines ☐

What are your own signals that depression (or some other unwanted mood state) might be trying to take hold again? Think back over your past experience and, as best you can, recall the patterns that might have given you early warning that your mood was slipping. Use the questions on the following pages as a guide; feel free to copy or download them from *www.guilford.com/teasdale-materials.*

Often other people may be aware of changes long before you register them yourself. If it feels comfortable, include ***someone you trust, who knows you well, and whom you see often*** in a collaborative effort to ***notice*** and then to ***respond*** rather than to ***react*** to these signs.

DEPRESSION EARLY WARNING SYSTEM

What triggers emotional distress or depression for you?

_____

_____

_____

_____

_____

_____

- Triggers can be external (things that happen to you) or internal (e.g., thoughts, feelings, memories, concerns).
- Consider small triggers as well as large ones—sometimes something that seems quite trivial can spark a downward mood spiral.

_____

_____

What sorts of thoughts run through your mind when you first feel your mood dropping or your feelings running out of control?

_____

_____

_____

_____

_____

What other emotions do you notice as well?

_____

_____

_____

_____

_____

What happens in your body?

_____

_____

_____

_____

_____

_____

What do you do or feel like doing?

_____

_____

_____

_____

_____

_____

What old habits of thinking or behavior might unwittingly keep you stuck in painful moods? (e.g., ruminating, trying to suppress or turn away from painful thoughts and feelings, struggling with them instead of allowing and exploring them)

_____

_____

_____

_____

_____

_____

What, in the past, has prevented you from noticing and attending to warning signs and signals? (e.g., pushing away, denial, distraction, a sense of hopelessness, using alcohol, arguments, blaming family members or colleagues)

_____

_____

_____

_____

_____

_____

How might you include friends and family members in your early warning system?

_____

_____

_____

_____

_____

_____

It's quite likely that thinking back to the past in this way has reawakened some sad feelings right now. If this is true for you, now would be a good time to

Take a 3-minute breathing space.

We'll be looking at what you can actually do once you detect early warning signs next week.

For now, you might like to create an "executive summary" of your exploration of warning signals by including the **most important five signals** in a description of your **Early Warning Signs** (Relapse Signature); feel free to copy or download from *www.guilford.com/teasdale-materials* the form on page 168.

MY EARLY WARNING SIGNS (RELAPSE SIGNATURE)

The five key signs that tell me that my life may be spinning out of control or that depression may be taking hold again are:

1. _____

_____

2. _____

_____

3. _____

_____

4. _____

_____

5. _____

_____

STEPPING BACK FROM THOUGHT

It is remarkable how liberating it feels to be able to see that your thoughts are just thoughts and not "you" or "reality." For instance, if you have the thought that you must get a certain number of things done today and you don't recognize it as a thought, but act as if it's "the truth," then you have created in that moment a reality in which you really believe that those things must all be done today.

One patient, Peter, who'd had a heart attack and wanted to prevent another one, came to a dramatic realization of this one night, when he found himself washing his car at 10 o'clock at night with the floodlights on in the driveway. It struck him that he didn't have to be doing this. It was just the inevitable result of a whole day spent trying to fit everything in that he thought needed doing today. As he saw what he was doing to himself, he also saw that he had been unable to question the truth of his original conviction that everything had to get done today, because he was already so completely caught up in believing it.

If you find yourself behaving in similar ways, it is likely that you will also feel driven, tense, and anxious without even knowing why, just as Peter did. So if the thought of how much you have to get done today comes up while you are meditating, you will have to be very attentive to it as a thought or you may be up and doing things before you know it, without any awareness that you decided to stop sitting simply because a thought came through your mind.

On the other hand, when such a thought comes up, if you are able to step back from it and see it clearly, you will be able to prioritize things and make sensible decisions about what really does need doing. You will know when to call it quits during the day. So the simple act of recognizing your thoughts as thoughts can free you from the distorted reality they often create and allow for more clear-sightedness and a greater sense of manageability in your life.

This liberation from the tyranny of the thinking mind comes directly out of the meditation practice itself. When we spend some time each day in a state of nondoing, observing the flow of the breath and the activity of our mind and body, without getting caught up in that activity, we are cultivating calmness and mindfulness hand in hand. As the mind develops stability and is less caught up in the content of thinking, we strengthen the mind's ability to concentrate and to be calm. And if each time we recognize a thought as a thought when it arises and register its content and discern the strength of its hold on us and the accuracy of its content, then each time we let go of it and come back to our breathing and a sense of our body, we are strengthening mindfulness. We come to know ourselves better and become more accepting of ourselves, not as we would like to be, but as we actually are.

JON KABAT-ZINN

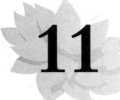

Week 7:
Kindness in Action

Orientation

Take a few moments to bring to mind what you do during a typical week.

In the spaces below, jot down 10 of the activities that make up your life at home or at work. An example has already been entered for you.

See if you can break down big chunks of activity—such as "work" or "housework"—into smaller parts, such as "talking to colleagues," "e-mails," "preparing meals," or "doing the laundry."

Activity 1 _Taking a shower_ _____

Activity 2 _____

Activity 3 _____

Activity 4 _____

Activity 5 _____

Activity 6 _____

Activity 7 _____

Activity 8 _____

Activity 9 _____

Activity 10 _____

Now, considering each of these activities in turn, ask yourself these two questions:

1. Does this activity lift my mood, give me energy, nourish me, or increase my sense of being alive? If the answer is "yes," put the letter N (for "nourishing") next to it.

2. Does this activity dampen my mood, drain me of energy, or decrease my sense of being alive? If the answer is "yes," put a D (for "depleting" or "draining") next to it.

Most likely, you will end up with some activities with Ns next to them, some with Ds next to them, and some with neither.

Although very simple, this exercise reminds us of something very important:

What you do affects how you feel. Most important:
You can change how you feel by changing what you do.

To make the most of this strategy, it's important to remember what "The Office" exercise (pages 149–150) revealed: the same event or activity can have very different effects on your feelings, depending on a host of other factors such as the mood you are already in, the meaning you give to the event, or unhelpful thoughts that can interfere.

Until we take account of these factors, the actions we take to lift mood will not necessarily have the effects we intend.

> I've tried to use activity to get rid of depression in the past, but I didn't find it very effective.

> You are not alone in this. It's quite subtle:
>
> 1. The <u>kind of activity</u> can make a big difference. Some activities are not so useful; others are more effective. Sometimes it's difficult to know beforehand.
>
> 2. The <u>intention</u> behind the activity is crucial—we'll come back to this later.
>
> 3. <u>Negative thinking</u> can really undermine activity: It's so difficult when we have an inner voice saying "There's no point—nothing will make a difference"; "I don't deserve to do things for myself"; "I don't get as much pleasure from things as I used to, so why bother?"
>
> MBCT addresses each of these potential problems. Read on!

The good news is that if you are actually present in the moment, and able to make mindful, informed decisions about what you really need:

You can turn activity into a simple yet powerful way to raise mood and enhance well-being.

Research has revealed the encouraging truth that skillful use of activity, by itself, can be an effective treatment for depression.

1. Activities That Help: Mastery and Pleasure

When people feel down, exhausted, and lacking energy, it turns out that two types of activities are particularly effective ways to lift mood:

1. **Pleasure** activities: these are things that give a sense of enjoyment or pleasure—like calling a friend for a chat, taking a long, hot, leisurely bath, or going for a walk.
2. **Mastery** activities: these are things that give a sense of accomplishment, satisfaction, or control—activities like writing a letter, mowing the lawn, doing something you've been putting off.

Mastery activities may not be pleasurable in themselves, but something in the world is different after doing them.

It's important to know there is a ***two-way relationship*** between mastery and pleasure activities and feeling down:

On the one hand, these activities can lift mood.

But:

On the other hand, as your mood gets lower and lower, you're likely to enjoy them less and you'll probably get less satisfaction from them than when your mood is more balanced.

It's then easy to think that these activities have little to offer. But, crucially:

Even when you're depressed, you can take advantage of the link between mood and mastery and pleasure activities. With care, you can tip the balance of the two-way relationship so that these activities will improve mood.

How do you do this?

Step 1 is to examine your day-to-day experience to discover the mastery and pleasure activities that are **already** in your life.

Having these tools **available in advance** means they are there for you when you need to use activity to cope with depression.

You might like, right now, to reflect on your own experience and begin to make a list of 10 pleasure (P) activities and 10 mastery (M) activities, using the forms on this page and the next.

It's fine to use activities you identified as Nourishing (**N**) in the earlier exercise—the important thing is to make a start (and you don't have to get all 10 right now!).

MY LIST OF PLEASURE (P) ACTIVITIES

Examples: *Visit a friend, watch something funny or uplifting on TV, listen to music, have a nice hot bath, treat yourself to a favorite food.*

P Activity 1 _____

P Activity 2 _____

P Activity 3 _____

P Activity 4 _____

P Activity 5 _____

P Activity 6 _____

P Activity 7 _____

P Activity 8 _____

P Activity 9 _____

P Activity 10 _____

MY LIST OF MASTERY (M) ACTIVITIES

Examples: *Clear out a drawer, pay a bill, catch up with e-mails, wash the car, do something you have put off doing (no matter how small or irrelevant it may seem).*

M Activity 1 _____

M Activity 2 _____

M Activity 3 _____

M Activity 4 _____

M Activity 5 _____

M Activity 6 _____

M Activity 7 _____

M Activity 8 _____

M Activity 9 _____

M Activity 10 _____

The **second step,** now that you've identified your list of M and P activities, is to weave them into the fabric of your life right now, while your mood is relatively good.

Building mastery and pleasure activities into your life *before* you get stressed out, exhausted, or depressed means:

1. They are there at your fingertips to lift mood as soon as you notice mood sinking. Having them already available means you are more likely to think of them and persist with them in the face of negative thoughts like, Why bother with anything?

2. Your everyday life will be happier and more satisfying.

Feel free to copy (or download from *www.guilford.com/teasdale-materials*) the forms so you have your lists with you.

Two Ways to Weave M and P Activities into Your Everyday Life

Strategy 1: Build the activity into your daily or weekly schedule.

For example, a very simple, proven way to take care of your mental and physical well-being is to take daily physical exercise—as a minimum, aim for at least one brisk, 10-minute walk a day (you might even do it mindfully!). Also, if at all possible, engage in other types of exercise, such as mindful stretching, yoga, swimming, jogging, and so on. Once exercise is in your regular routine, it's there to turn to as a response to depressed moods as they arise.

Strategy 2: Link M and P activities to Responsive 3-Minute Breathing Spaces.

The breathing space provides a way to remind us to use activity to deal with unpleasant feelings as they arise. We'll describe this strategy fully when we get to Daily Practice.

2. Intention Is Key

Years of experience with using activity to respond skillfully to depression and states of low energy suggests two aspects of intention are pivotal.

We give these details here so you can see if you recognize the same patterns in your own experience:

In Depression Motivation Works Backwards

How things work differently in depression:

1. When you're not depressed: You can wait until you want to do something before you actually do it.

   In depression, you have to do something *before* you're able to want to do it.

Hint: It's best not to wait until you *feel* like doing something before actually doing it—see if it's possible, instead, to do it anyway and see what you discover.

2. When you're not depressed, if you're tired, rest can refresh you.

   When you're depressed, resting can actually *increase* tiredness.

Hint: It's best not to give up on activities to rest whenever you feel fatigued—see if it's possible, instead, to "stay in the game"—carrying on with activities, perhaps even briefly increasing activity—even if your mood and thoughts seem to say "no."

Joshua: "This is the one most important thing I learned in the MBCT course: When I feel down, I remember the words 'In depression, things work backwards.'

"Other mottos I now use are:

'I don't have to like it; I just have to do it.'

'It is no good waiting until I feel better to try to sort things out. It doesn't work that way.'

"Even kindergarten motivational techniques, if they work, are good for me. I got a large project finished by asking my partner to put a gold star on a chart if I had done 30 hours' work on the project during the week (I was also working part-time on another project at the time). Small thing—but it really helped.

"I used to think I was being stupid to use such techniques. Then I remembered something someone said in another context: 'If it's stupid and it works, it ain't stupid.'"

Katarina was an avid film buff. But since she had become depressed she had stopped going to the movies. With thoughts like "I am just not interested," "I'll just feel awkward and alone," and "I'd rather wait until I can enjoy going out again," her motivation was never strong enough to get her out of the house.

Through mindfulness practice, Katarina came to see the difference between her moment-to-moment experience and how her thoughts represented things. This was especially clear one time when she was working with painful sensations in her shoulder. Her thoughts told her the pain was unbearable—but she found she *could* manage to bear the sensations by breathing into them and out from them.

Using this as an analogy, she decided to suspend her beliefs and go see a movie. She reported that while feeling a bit uneasy at first, the story gradually drew her in and she felt good about returning to what used to be a comfortable routine.

The film didn't have an immediate impact on Katarina's mood, but it did engage her more than she had anticipated. As a result, Katarina began to schedule weekly activities and to follow through, regardless of whether she felt motivated to do them. By being willing to experiment with the idea that, in depression, motivation works backward, Katarina allowed the impact of her activities to rebuild her motivation and help her slowly regain her active life.

Kindness Heals; Unkindness (Aversion) Hinders

Have a look at the following two scenarios:

SCENARIO 1

Tom: "Last night I got home, and as I stepped through the door into my empty apartment a wave of sadness and weariness swept over me. I could feel my mood sinking fast. Then I recalled that activity is a way to get rid of depression. I thought of my list of M and P activities and chose listening to my favorite music as the one most likely to shift my mood. I put on the music and settled down to listen. But, as I listened, I found myself wondering, 'Is it working? Is the sadness going away yet?' and I found myself focusing on my mood rather than the music. I had to keep forcing my attention back to the music—but then I was irritated with myself and frustrated that the music wasn't working. In the end, I just had to call it quits—if anything I felt worse rather than better, and that left me with a sense of dissatisfaction that lasted the whole evening. I was glad to get to bed and blank it all out."

SCENARIO 2

Jim: "Last night I got home, and as I stepped through the door into my empty apartment a wave of sadness and weariness swept over me. I could feel my mood sinking fast. Then I recalled that activity is a way to look after myself. I thought of my list of M and P activities and asked myself '<u>How can I best take care of myself right now?</u>' I chose listening to my favorite music as a way to treat myself kindly, to give myself a little treat, in that moment. I put on the music, made myself physically comfortable, and settled down to listen. My mind drifted away from time to time, but, as best I could, I treated myself gently. I could feel the relief in my mind and body as they sensed they were getting some kindly attention at last. Thoughts of other ways in which I could take it easy that evening came to mind. When the music stopped, I noticed the sadness and weariness had lifted a little. I puttered about the rest of the evening, quite pleasantly, until it was time for bed."

In these two scenarios we have the same activity—"listening to my favorite music"—with very different outcomes produced by different intentions.

The negative aversive intention—Tom using the music with the aim of **getting rid** of the sadness and sinking mood (shown in the way he kept checking to see if his mood was improving)—just fueled more aversion and unpleasant feelings.

The positive kindly intention—Jim using the music as a way to **take care** of himself when he felt sad and low—enabled healing to occur.

How you use mastery and pleasure activities (the spirit or intention behind them) is more important than *what* you do.

As best you can, see if it's possible to engage in mastery or pleasure activities as an act of kindness to yourself.

When you feel low in spirits, drained, with all your energy going or gone, take your time to ask yourself: "How can I best take care of myself right now?"

3. Thoughts That Stand in the Way

"There are things in life over which you don't have a choice, like going to work."

"I wasn't raised to take time for myself."

"My parents are elderly and need caring for. It would be wrong for me to put myself first."

"You can only do something nice for yourself once your obligations to others, or to your work, have been satisfied."

"I'm balancing being a mom, a career woman, a wife, and a housekeeper. Where do I find the time for myself?"

Thoughts such as these, with themes of hopelessness ("It's all too difficult"), coupled with guilt about taking more time for yourself, are likely to undermine your motivation to engage in actions that could be effective in increasing your well-being.

So what can you do?

Jackie was a nurse on a busy hospital ward, always, as she said, "being knocked off her feet" with one thing after another. There simply seemed to be no time for her to relax, far less to sit and meditate. But she started to pay more attention within the busyness. She noticed that little spaces opened up even at the most hectic times. She said, for example, that she had needed to phone someone in another part of the hospital to get some test results on a patient. She phoned several times but got no reply. This was one of the most frustrating aspects of her job, waiting for someone in another department to answer the phone when she had so much to do. She had started to get angry and to criticize herself for getting frustrated so easily.

Then she stopped. Here was 30 seconds in which she could not rush around; here was a moment of potential silence in the noise of the day. She started to use the lack of an answer as an opportunity to take a breathing space, to step back. Gradually she started to notice many other times when she could step back; for example, pushing a medication cart, which limited the pace of movement along the corridor, or walking to the other end of the ward to see a patient's family. Prior to this, she had thought that meditation practice might best be done when taking a lunch break or going to the rest room. Now she found she could look for the in-between spaces throughout the day, spaces that transformed her thoughts, feelings, and behavior for the rest of the activities of the day.

Mindfulness practice helped Jackie:

1. "turn toward" rather than escape or avoid her experience
2. see thoughts *as thoughts*—not to take at face value the thoughts that told her she was stupid to be frustrated.

Together these two critically important shifts in the way she approached things allowed Jackie to engage creatively with her situation—to find the spaces in the busyness where she could take time for herself even within her hectic, demanding life.

The Responsive 3-Minute Breathing Space offers a way for you to do the same in your own life. It is a major focus of Daily Practice this week.

Daily Practice

During Week 7, practice in these ways **for 6 out of the next 7 days**:

1. Sustainable Mindfulness Practice
2. 3-Minute Breathing Space—Regular
3. 3-Minute Breathing Space—Responsive: The Door of Mindful Action

In addition:

4. Prepare an Action Plan

1. Sustainable Mindfulness Practice

From the various forms of formal mindfulness practice you have explored (body scan, sitting meditations of varying lengths and types, mindful stretching, mindful movement, mindful walking, regular 3-minute breathing spaces), see if it's possible to settle on a pattern of practice that you can **realistically sustain** once the 8 weeks of the program are over.

It's fine to have different daily practices for weekdays and on the weekend. The vital thing is that you acknowledge the real constraints on your time while honoring mindfulness practice as a really important source of daily nourishment for you.

> As best you can, find a pattern of practice you feel comfortable with—there's no need to force yourself to heroic efforts that are not sustainable. It's better to plan too little (you can always add more later!) than plan too much (which may lead you to give up altogether).

Each day, jot down what you intended to do, what you actually did, and what you learned about how workable that level of practice was.

At the end of the week, there will be an opportunity for you to finalize the pattern of practice you intend to follow over the long term.

MY PRACTICES FOR THE WEEK

Day 1:
Intended practice:

_____

Actual practice:

_____

I learned:

_____

Day 2:
Intended practice:

_____

Actual practice:

_____

I learned:

_____

Day 3:
Intended practice:

_____

Actual practice:

_____

I learned:

_____

Day 4:
Intended practice:

_____

Actual practice:

_____

I learned:

_____

Day 5:
Intended practice:

_____

Actual practice:

_____

I learned:

_____

Day 6:
Intended practice:

_____

Actual practice:

_____

I learned:

_____

At the end of the week, take some time to look over and reflect on what you noted each day. Then see if it's possible to put down in writing the pattern of formal practice you intend to sustain from now on. The box below has spaces where you can jot down different patterns for weekdays and the weekend, but feel free to use the same pattern for both if that feels more comfortable. If you like, you can copy the form for later use or download it from *www.guilford.com/teasdale-materials*.

We have already written in *Responsive Breathing Spaces* as a reminder that we recommend that this **always** be your first response to any awareness of difficult or unpleasant feelings.

My Pattern of Daily Practice

Weekdays:

1. _Responsive Breathing Spaces_

2. _____

3. _____

Weekend:

1. _Responsive Breathing Spaces_

2. _____

3. _____

From *The Mindful Way Workbook*. Copyright 2014 by The Guilford Press.

---

2. The 3-Minute Breathing Space—Regular

Every day this week, take a 3-minute breathing space three times a day, at the times you have decided in advance, just as you did last week.

To keep track of your practice, at the end of each day, circle an **R** in the next table for each of these planned breathing spaces you take.

Day 1	R R R	Day 4	R R R
Day 2	R R R	Day 5	R R R
Day 3	R R R	Day 6	R R R

3. The 3-Minute Breathing Space—Responsive: The Door of Mindful Action

Last week we introduced the image of the responsive breathing space taking us into a hall out of which three doors—**re-entry, body, thoughts**—offered us different options for what to do next.

This week we introduce another door—the Door of Mindful Action.

THE BREATHING SPACE: THE DOOR OF MINDFUL ACTION

As you come to the end of a responsive breathing space, after reconnecting with an expanded awareness in the third step, it may feel appropriate to take some **considered action**.

Ask yourself: *What do I need for myself right now? How can I best take care of myself right now?*

In responding to depressed feelings, the following activities may be particularly helpful:

1. **Do something pleasurable.** Choose an activity from your list of P (pleasure) activities (page 173) or use any other pleasurable activity that is at hand or seems appropriate.

2. **Do something that gives you a sense of mastery, satisfaction, achievement, or control.** Choose an activity from your list of M (mastery) activities (page 174) or use any other mastery activity that is at hand or seems appropriate. Remember (a) to break tasks down into smaller steps or chunks and tackle only one step at a time and (b) to take a moment to really appreciate your efforts whenever you complete a task or part of a task.

3. **Act mindfully** (read Staying Present, page 185). As best you can, focus your attention on just what you are doing right now; let your mind rest in this very moment, paying attention particularly to the sensations in your body. You may find it helpful to softly describe your actions to yourself (e.g., "Now I am walking down the stairs . . . now I can feel the banister beneath my hand . . . now I'm walking into the kitchen . . . now I'm turning on the light . . ."); be aware of your breathing as you do other things; be aware of the contact of your feet with the floor as you walk.

Remember

1. As best you can, perform your action as an experiment. See if it's possible to let go of the tendency to prejudge how you'll feel after it's completed. Keep an open mind about whether doing this will be helpful in any way.

2. Consider a range of activities and don't limit yourself to a favorite few.

> Sometimes trying new behaviors can be interesting in itself. "Exploring" and "inquiring" often work against "withdrawal" and "retreat."
>
> 3. Don't expect miracles. Carry out what you've planned as best you can. Putting extra pressure on yourself by expecting this to alter things dramatically may be unrealistic. Rather, activities are helpful in building your overall sense of control in the face of shifts in your mood.
>
> 4. There's no need to wait until you *feel* like doing an activity—just do it!

Every day this week, in addition to the planned Regular Breathing Space, take a breathing space *whenever you notice any unpleasant feelings,* and, **at least once a day,** explore using the **Action Door,** using the suggestions on page 183 for guidance.

Each day, keep track of your experience with this new door (**What was the situation? What did you do? What happened?**) by jotting down a few notes:

Day 1:

Situation: _____

_____

Action: _____

_____

Outcome: _____

_____

> It was midafternoon at work, I was getting tired, and I could feel a heaviness growing. I wondered what I could do about it, but the thoughts I had— "go shopping," "see a friend"—were unrealistic. So I took a breathing space—not the full 3 minutes, maybe a minute altogether—and asked myself, "How can I best take care of myself right now?" And up popped an answer: "mindful coffee." I "gifted" myself, as an act of kindness, five minutes in which I <u>really</u> focused on the experience of drinking a cup of coffee—a bit like eating the raisin. And I returned to work a little more at ease, more spacious in my mind, refreshed.

> Wonderful! A slight shift in feeling is often enough to let us "start again" from a different place. Then we may not go down the same old grooves, but we can allow life to unfold in new and different ways.

Staying Present

Remember to use your body as a way to awareness. It can be as simple as staying mindful of your posture. You are probably sitting as you read this. What are the sensations in your body at this moment? When you finish reading and stand, feel the movements of standing, of walking to the next activity, of how you lie down at the end of the day. Be in your body as you move, as you reach for something, as you turn. It is as simple as that.

Just patiently practice feeling what is there—and the body is always there—until it becomes second nature to know even the small movements you make. If you are reaching for something, you are doing it anyway; there is nothing extra you have to do. Simply notice the reaching. You are moving. Can you train yourself to be there, to feel it?

It is very simple. Practice again and again bringing your attention back to your body. This basic effort, which, paradoxically, is a relaxing back into the moment, gives us the key to expanding our awareness from times of formal meditation to living mindfully in the world. Do not underestimate the power that comes to you from feeling the simple movements of your body throughout the day.

JOSPEH GOLDSTEIN

Day 2:

Situation: _____

_____

Action: _____

_____

Outcome: _____

_____

I felt burdened and exhausted by all the things I had to do, so the idea of doing something to feel mastery or pleasure seemed like yet another thing on my "to do" list. But I took a breathing space anyway and asked myself, "What do I need for myself right now?" I got this very clear sense of needing a break, peace, some time for myself. But I knew that just lying on the couch would lead to rumination, so I chose to "rest" in simple movements of the body. I ended up just mindfully walking up and down, very slowly, very gently—it was quite peaceful and restful. It felt good to give myself some care for a change.

That's a lovely example of using the breathing space with an open mind—to end up doing something you hadn't expected but that turned out to be just what you needed. Great!

Day 3:

Situation: _____

_____

Action: _____

_____

Outcome: _____

_____

I'd taken a breathing space, opened the Action Door, and decided "Mastery activity: mow the lawn," something I've been putting off. To keep the job manageable, I was aiming just to do the smaller of my two lawns. It didn't take long, and I felt pleased that I'd done it. And then the nagging voice in my head got on the case: "That's not much. Shouldn't you do the big one as well?" I sighed a little, shrugged my shoulders, and was just about to start again when I remembered, This is meant to be about taking care of myself. So I was kind! I put the mower away and went and put my feet up. It felt like a small triumph.

That's such an important thing you did! Every time you are kind to yourself in the face of the "shoulds," "oughts," and "musts," you sow the seeds of a new way of being.

Remember to tell yourself "well done"
whenever you complete a task or part of a task.

It can really help to **break an activity down
into smaller, more manageable steps**.

You could break it up either by time (doing something for
only a few minutes, then giving yourself permission to stop)
or by activity (doing only one aspect of a larger activity, such
as clearing one part of a desk rather than the whole desk),
and, after each step, pause to appreciate what you've done.

Day 4:

Situation: _____

_____

Action: _____

_____

Outcome: _____

_____

I'm still not sure why I need to do the breathing space first. Wouldn't it be simpler just to get on with an M or P activity right away?

This is something you can check out for yourself by experimenting with taking action with and without a breathing space. We recommend always starting with a breathing space because, that way, your action is born from being mode rather than doing mode. This means actions are more likely to spring from kindness than from aversion, to be more creative, reflecting a bigger picture of the situation, and you'll be more likely to see blocking thoughts <u>as</u> thoughts. And, of course, after a breathing space you may find it's more appropriate to open a different door altogether and leave the action door for another time.

The breathing space is helpful because
it links us to the wider aspects of the program—
it "brings all its friends to the party"
(in the shape of reminders of everything you've learned).

Day 5:

Situation: _____

_____

Action: _____

_____

Outcome: _____

_____

I'd been feeling down for a while and gotten into the habit of not seeing my friends—it just felt like too much effort, and I thought I wouldn't enjoy it and they would find me boring. Then a few of them invited me out for a meal. The usual thoughts went through my mind, and I was at the point of finding some excuse when I saw a supermarket delivery truck with the logo "Do something different today!" in bright orange letters. So I took a breathing space, opened the Thought Door, remembered "Thoughts aren't facts," and went on to open the Action Door. I ended up joining my friends—it wasn't easy, but they were so glad to see me I was really glad I'd made the effort.

There are times that taking action is the most important thing: simply having the courage to do something that you don't feel like doing may be what your body and mind need most.

Day 6:

Situation: _____

_____

Action: _____

_____

Outcome: _____

_____

It was the weekend, I was alone, it was cold and raining out, and I was feeling miserable. I wondered about doing something useful, but it all seemed too much effort, so I took a rest on the sofa, which didn't help at all. Finally I got around to a breathing space and chose the Action Door. I sensed the need to move my body, but the idea of a walk in the rain did not appeal. But from somewhere came a reminder: "In depression motivation works backwards—just do it!" So I did, and, you know, I actually enjoyed it—the wind in my hair, the rain on my skin woke me up, and the walking itself seemed to clear my mind. I walked for 30 minutes, then called a friend to meet up.

It's helpful to remember that low mood affects the <u>body</u> as well as thoughts and feelings—physical exercise can have surprisingly powerful effects in lifting mood.

Getting the body active can reverse
the fatigue and inertia of depressed mood.

4. Preparing an Action Plan

Last week you identified your early warning signs—the pattern of signals that will alert you (and those around you) that things are beginning to deteriorate and it is time to take constructive action.

This week the aim is to develop a specific concrete plan for what you will actually do.

See if it's possible to involve friends and family so you can work together to develop your action plan and put it into practice at times of need.

How might you respond most skillfully when you notice early warning signs?

You may find it helpful to reflect on your experience over the years, as well as looking back over your entries in this workbook. Both can be really good ways to remind you of what you have done and what you have discovered that is helpful.

In the past, what has helped you when you were starting to feel bad?

_____

_____

_____

_____

_____

_____

_____

_____

_____

What might be a skillful response to the mental pain or low mood you're feeling? How could you respond best to the turmoil of thoughts and feelings without adding to it (including what you have learned in this course)?

_____

_____

_____

_____

_____

_____

_____

_____

_____

_____

How can you best take care of yourself at this difficult and painful time (e.g., things that would soothe you, activities that might nourish you, people you might contact, small things you could do to respond wisely to your distress)?

_____

_____

_____

_____

_____

_____

_____

_____

_____

In the past, *what obstacles* have stopped you from taking useful steps to help yourself when things were beginning to get out of hand? How might you deal with these obstacles if they were to arise in the future?

_____

_____

_____

_____

_____

_____

_____

_____

_____

On page 193, you are invited to summarize what you have learned from making these notes, as well as from last week's notes on early warning signs, into specific suggestions for an *action plan*—something you can use as a framework for coping, once you, or your friends or family, notice early warning signs.

You may find it helpful to write this in the form of a kindly letter to yourself, as if you were writing to a dear friend in difficulty—in that spirit, we have suggested a beginning for you: "I know you probably will not be keen on this idea, but I think it is very important for you to. . . . "

You may find this structure helpful:

- **Step 1:** Always begin with a **breathing space**—we've written this in for you.

- **Step 2:** Choose a practice you've found helpful in the past to **gather yourself as best you can** (e.g., put on a mindful movement, body scan, or sitting meditation audio; remind yourself of what you have learned in the course that was helpful then; take frequent breathing spaces leading into thought review; read something that will "reconnect" you with your "wiser" mind).

- **Step 3: Take some action** that will give a sense of *pleasure* or *mastery* (e.g., from your lists of P and M activities), even if it seems futile to do so. Break activities down into smaller parts (e.g., doing only part of a task or doing it for only a short, easily managed period of time).

What you need at times of difficulty
is no different from what you have already practiced
many times throughout this course.

My Action Plan

Dear _____:

I know you probably will not be keen on this idea, but I think it is very important for you to take action as soon as you or those around you notice the following signs that tell you that things are beginning to get out of control:

1. _____   2. _____

3. _____   4. _____

5. _____

I recommend the following action:

- **Step 1:** Begin with a breathing space.
- **Step 2:** Use these practices to gather yourself as best you can:

    _____

    _____

    _____

- **Step 3:** Take some action that will give a sense of **pleasure** or **mastery:**

    _____

    _____

    _____

Be **mindful** of the following obstacles that may block constructive action:

_____

_____

_____

What you need at this time is no different from what you have already practiced many times throughout the MBCT course.

Good luck!

Signed _____ Date _____

Feel free, if it feels comfortable, to photocopy and share this plan with friends and family. The blank form can be found at *www.guilford.com/teasdale-materials*.

When Feelings Seem Overwhelming

Most likely, there will come days when your feelings overwhelm you so rapidly that it feels impossible to do anything about it.

At such times, it's vital to remember that, even then, there ***are*** things you can do to make a difference—the most important thing is to reconnect with some sense of control, however slight that may be.

> If you can improve mood in this moment by 1%, you have made an enormously important shift: the quality of this moment affects the next moment, which affects the next, and so on, and on . . .

One small change can have a large impact in the end.

Steve: "I have, at various times, had to take time off work because of work-related stress and depression, including the entire second half of one year a few years back. I have used much of the range of treatments available for depression, including medication, cognitive therapy (CT), and MBCT—particularly the body scan. When I feel really bad, I feel really useless—and that it will go on forever. One of my unhelpful approaches when I was really depressed was to think that staying longer and longer after work was the way to get things done. It wasn't. It is a way to spend longer and longer getting less and less done, in the environment that probably depressed me most at that moment.

"At these times, I'm not able to develop a comprehensive 'getting everything done' strategy, and if I could I would be in no shape to do it even if I wrote it all down.

"At these times, my strategy is this: 'Steve—do anything, anything at all.' I find that ANYTHING that is marginally useful will get the ball rolling and help me feel better. It can be really small, but it is really important to do something, and, if I can, I involve a close, trusted colleague. It might be that, a moment ago, I was thinking, I will never be able to do anything useful ever again. But then, if I DO something—even if it is only to throw away three old newspapers—I have proved that the total, crushing belief is not true."

The Summer Day

Who made the world?
Who made the swan, and the black bear?
Who made the grasshopper?
This grasshopper, I mean—
the one who has flung herself out of the grass,
the one who is eating sugar out of my hand,
who is moving her jaws back and forth instead of up and down—
who is gazing around with her enormous and complicated eyes.
Now she lifts her pale forearms and thoroughly washes her face.
Now she snaps her wings open, and floats away.
I don't know exactly what a prayer is.
I do know how to pay attention, how to fall down
into the grass, how to kneel down in the grass,
how to be idle and blessed, how to stroll through the fields,
which is what I have been doing all day.
Tell me, what else should I have done?
Doesn't everything die at last, and too soon?
Tell me, what is it you plan to do
with your one wild and precious life?

MARY OLIVER

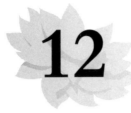

12

Week 8:
What Now?

Orientation

What is it you plan to do with your one wild and precious life?

How will you respond to this vital question posed by Mary Oliver in her poem (page 195)?

How might the MBCT program help you realize your heart's deepest wish for greater happiness, wholeness, satisfaction, and well-being?

People vary widely in what they find most valuable in MBCT. Here are some of the things previous participants have said:

"I'm less cross and angry with my 18-year-old daughter. I'm able to relate to her more constructively."

"I now have tactics when I sense a low mood or depression starting."

"If I take something on, I feel I've got the resources, instead of always being afraid it would collapse. I'm starting to think I could manage."

"It has removed the shame I felt about having been depressed and anxious in the past, leading to greater self-acceptance."

"There were emotions I had been repressing for years. To really live my life, I had to feel them. My whole perspective on life has changed."

"I have discovered an inner strength."

It's quite possible that much of what you have gained from the time and effort you've invested in your practice may not be obvious to you right now.

In Week 8 there is a chance to reflect on your own experience with the program: *What have you experienced? What have you learned? What have you valued most?*

Actually putting into words what you have discovered can remind, inspire, and reinspire you as you consider how to take forward into the rest of your life the fruits of your patience and persistence over these last weeks.

Might it be that Week 8 marks not so much the end of the program as the beginning of a much wider continuing journey of mindful discovery?

> The real Week 8 is the rest of our lives.
>
> JON KABAT-ZINN

When we teach MBCT in a class, at this point we come full circle and do a body scan—the first extended practice of the program from Week 1.

If you are not in a class, you might like to do the same right now, re-entering the mode of being before continuing to reflect further on your experience of the program as a whole. Feel free to do this with or without the guiding voice of the CD or audio downloads that accompany this book.

What do you notice? How was your experience the same or different from that of Week 1? (You might like to look back at the notes you made then.) Make a note of any similarities and contrasts.

And as you stand back now, to reflect more widely on your experience of the course as a whole, you might find it helpful to bear in mind these two interlinked overarching aims of MBCT:

Aim 1: to help you recognize earlier and respond more skillfully to the habitual patterns of mind that create emotional distress and entangle you in persistent emotional suffering

Aim 2: to cultivate a new way of being:

- a way of being that means that destructive habitual patterns of mind are less likely to be triggered
- a way of being that allows you to live all of life with greater well-being, ease, and satisfaction
- a way of being that is more ready to trust the mind's inner wisdom to guide you, with kindness, through emotional turmoil

What do other people find most helpful in MBCT? Here, below, are some of the themes that come up most often in what participants tell us.

How important have these been for you?

Give a score from 1 through 10 where 1 means not at all important, 10 means extremely important.

Theme	Score (1–10)
Knowing what pulls mood down and recognizing early warning signs	_____
Learning new ways to step out of patterns of negative thoughts and feelings	_____
Seeing negative thoughts and feelings differently—as parts of emotional packages, not "me"	_____
Feeling less helpless in the face of unwanted emotions	_____
Feeling less alone—seeing that many other people experience depression or other difficult emotions and that it is not "just me"	_____
Being kinder and less critical to myself	_____
Valuing myself more—recognizing and meeting my own needs	_____

Another way to reflect on your experience is to think back to the core features of the being mode of mind (pages 22–25) and to rate how important each of these features is to you now, using the same 1–10 scale:

Living with awareness and conscious choice (*versus* on "automatic pilot")   _____

Knowing experience directly through the senses (*versus* through thinking)   _____

Being here, now, in this moment (*versus* dwelling in the past or future)   _____

Approaching <u>all</u> experience with interest (*versus* avoiding the unpleasant)   _____

Allowing things to be as they are (*versus* <u>needing</u> them to be different)   _____

Seeing thoughts as mental events (*versus* as necessarily true and real)   _____

Taking care of yourself with kindness and compassion (*versus* focusing on achieving goals regardless of the cost to you or others)   _____

Jot down here any important ways that you feel you have benefited from MBCT so far (including little hints of important change, even if they have not yet had a chance to show themselves fully):

_____

_____

_____

_____

_____

_____

_____

_____

_____

Joanne: *"I am truly grateful for the experience of mindfulness you have given me. Mindfulness is having a quietly profound impact on me. I think it is working quietly beneath the surface.*

"I notice now that I can seize the moment with my children and bury myself in what we are doing together, rather than living in my thoughts about the day at work. I observe and follow their lead. I notice my boredom or irritation and can see that it is no different from the way my mind wanders in meditation—that is, that my mind has moved on to an adult task or pressure and I cease to attend fully to being with them.

"Sometimes attending to a feeling or a thought or sound can take me back to an intensity of feeling and I can recall, for the first time in years, sensations of the wind on my face as a child, clouds over my house at home, and feel again the total physical and emotional energy of youthful optimism and joy, of great possibilities, of a world to be discovered. This is a welcome surprise to me."

> By reflecting on the benefits you have gained
> from practicing mindfulness, you sow seeds of good intention
> that will support your practice in the future.

Looking Forward

At this point, there are two vital questions to consider:

1. **Why** might I wish to continue with some form of mindfulness practice?
2. **What** form might that practice take?

Let's first consider **why**.

Why Continue to Practice?

Do I really need to continue? I've put in a lot of time and effort for 8 weeks. I was hoping that was it!

That's very understandable—and, most likely, your life would be different and better even if you did no further formal mindfulness practice.

BUT all the evidence we have suggests that the people who benefit most from MBCT in the long run are the ones who keep going with some form of mindfulness practice—even if it's for only a few minutes a day.

To enjoy the full benefits from the time and effort you've already invested, it's helpful to remember that, just like learning a new language, <u>a little practice keeps a new skill alive and available</u>.

I don't know why I should do any practice or be mindful if I don't feel like it sometimes. If there's one thing I've learned, it's that "shoulds" are part of doing mode.

Absolutely—our experience with others suggests that "shoulds" won't keep your practice going for long. The skillful alternative is to identify some POSITIVE REASON that will help sustain your practice—to give you the motivation to do it whether you feel like it or not. Is it possible to link the intention for continuing to practice with something about which you already care deeply?

Giving yourself a positive reason to sustain mindfulness practice, linked to something about which you care deeply, can be enormously empowering.

IDENTIFYING A HEARTFELT INTENTION TO SUSTAIN MINDFULNESS PRACTICE

You may find this exercise helpful:

Settle down in a comfortable, relaxed, sitting position; take a few mindful breaths to gather your mind, and, if it feels comfortable, allow your eyes to close.

Allow the following question to drop gently into your mind and heart and to be held there softly in awareness:

> *"What is most important to me in my life [what do I most value] that the practice might help with?"*

Allow the question to drop into your mind as a smooth round pebble might fall down a deep well, or slowly, deeper and deeper, through the cool clear waters of a lake. . . . As the pebble falls, continue to hold the question in awareness. . . . An answer may arise in your mind, or it may not.

As the pebble reaches the bottom, allow it to rest there for a while, open to any further responses that enter awareness.

There's no need to think about the question or to try to puzzle out the answer or to look for a quick response. Instead, see if it's possible to let awareness respond in its own way, in its own time, allowing the depths of your being to process the question at a level beyond the usual thinking mind.

It's quite possible that when you first contemplate the question no answer will arise or the answer that arises will feel "not quite right" in some way. Remember that this is something you can always return to later.

When you are ready, take a slightly deeper breath and gently open your eyes.

**If you discovered a reason to practice mindfulness
that connects with something about which you care deeply,
note it below so that it is there whenever
you need it—to remind, reinspire, and reconnect you
with your heartfelt reason to practice.**

As best I can, I intend to continue to practice because:

_____

_____

_____

_____

_____

_____

_____

_____

Joanne: "I intend to keep practicing some form of mindfulness every day because mindfulness helps me feel closer to my children, and that is something I care about very deeply. During the weeks of the course, I seemed to have more time for them, I was sort of more available to them—and I enjoyed being with them so much more. It's funny, because early on I was worried that the time I had to spend on daily practice would take me away from my kids and my husband, but, in fact, just the opposite occurred—I feel closer to them now than I have in a long time."

Cary: "I value being in nature, so bringing that sense of seeing the leaves on the trees and feeling the wind in my hair . . . I used to take the dog for a walk but never noticed anything around me; it just became a task to get done . . . now I can feel quite joyous. That's what I care about."

Mo: "I value my physical and mental health. I can see the link between that and mindfulness—it helps me remember to do the yoga and the walking meditation and to check out what in my life nourishes me and what depletes me."

Clear intention is what carries us through, so that
we practice whether we feel like it or not—not by forcing
ourselves, but by reminding us of what we truly value.

In truth, we all already have within us a deeply rooted motivation that can sustain our practice and support us to act when painful emotions arise.

It is the simple, precious birthright we all share *to care about people—including ourselves.*

Of course, if you have been depressed in the past, or you are depressed now, it can be very hard to recognize or honor the intention to care for *yourself.* You may feel that you don't deserve to be cared for, or you may believe that, unlike everyone else, you just don't have this innate capacity to care.

At times like this, it's vital to remember that, just like everything else you've been exploring in MBCT, the intention to care, or to be kind, can be cultivated, nurtured, and strengthened by practice.

How? By bringing a mindful, allowing, interested awareness to your experience, to the extent you can, however much that may be. That action, itself, is a powerful gesture of care, goodwill, and kindness.

> *Every time we are truly mindful, we nourish the precious intention to care for ourselves and for other people.*

Of course, even with the best of intentions to practice, you'll probably encounter blocks and obstacles. But that doesn't mean those obstacles have to keep you stuck.

From past experience, what do you anticipate will be your biggest blocks or obstacles to continuing with mindfulness practice?

_____

_____

_____

_____

_____

From past experience, what strategies might help you get around those obstacles?

_____

_____

_____

_____

_____

The "What" of Continuing Practice: Daily Practice

Here are different ways to deepen your mindful way of living day by day:

1. Some Daily Formal Mindfulness Practice
2. Some Everyday Informal Mindfulness Practice
3. Plus 3-Minute Breathing Spaces—Responsive

1. Some Daily Formal Mindfulness Practice

As much as you possibly can, continue with the sustainable pattern of daily formal practice you settled on last week (page 182).

It may well be that you'll find you need to make some changes to that pattern in the light of future experience. That's fine—the important thing is that the pattern be sustainable on a daily basis, long term.

You may find it helpful to review your pattern of daily practice every 3 months or so, adjusting it as necessary. Entering the intention to review in your diary on a date 3 months from now can be a helpful reminder.

Lexy: "Toward the end of the MBCT course I was worried about incorporating mindfulness into my everyday life. I decided to spend a bit of time with my diary to work out times that I could put aside for the mindfulness exercises.

"Initially, I would stick to these times. However, as time went on, I found that the exercises became a natural part of my daily routine. I normally start the day with 10–15 minutes of either a body scan or a sitting meditation. I use the breathing space most days, usually when I am traveling to and from work. It's especially useful for stressful times during the day. For the longer meditation practices, I rely less and less on the CD.

"I think that everyday mindfulness is a fantastic concept. I simply go about my tasks and activities for the day as normal, but choose to do them mindfully.

"The MBCT course is brilliant in that it teaches a number of different mindfulness techniques, giving you choices about which ones fit best into your life.

"I have now been practicing mindfulness for approximately 2 years and have noticed some really positive changes. Before reacting to a situation, I can ground myself in that moment. I feel more in touch with how I am feeling physically and emotionally. Generally it has had a hugely calming effect on me and transformed my outlook on life."

Some Tips That Other Participants Found Helpful in Sustaining a Daily Formal Mindfulness Practice

- **Do some practice, no matter how brief, every day.** The "everydayness" of practice is hugely important as a way to keep mindfulness fresh, available, ready for you whenever you need it most—because you never know when that will be!

- Internationally respected meditation teacher Joseph Goldstein recommends that his students sit down to meditate every day—***even if only for 10 seconds.*** Experience suggests that, most often, those 10 seconds will be enough to encourage you to sit longer.

- **If at all possible, do the practice at the same time, in the same place, each day.** That way mindfulness gets built into the very fabric of your daily routine. Then, just as with brushing your teeth, you don't have to ponder whether to do it or not—you do it because that's what you always do at that point in your routine.

- **View practice like caring for a plant.** Give it a little water each day rather than a bucketful every month! Just as with a plant, nurturing your practice with consistent care and attention will allow it to grow and its natural potential for loveliness to unfold.

- **See practice as a way to nourish yourself, rather than another thing on your "to do" list.** Remember that the practice won't always *feel* nourishing—as much as you can, let the practice *be as it is*, letting go of your ideas of how *it should be* or of regarding it as part of a "project" of self-improvement.

- **Explore ways to inspire and reinspire yourself to practice.** Reread this workbook from time to time. Read other related books or listen to talks and guided meditations on the Internet (see the Resources section for suggestions).

- **Explore ways to practice with other people.** Practicing regularly with others—in what is often called a "sitting group"—is one of the most powerful ways to keep your practice vital and alive. If you learned MBCT with a group, look out for opportunities for reunions and practice days. Everyone can benefit from finding a mindfulness "buddy" with whom to practice and share experiences from time to time. *Even if it's only one person, joining with others to practice and share experiences is hugely, and often surprisingly, supportive.*

- **Remember, you can always begin again.** The essence of mindfulness practice is letting go of the past and starting afresh in each new moment (as you've already practiced many, many times in coming back to the breath when the mind has wandered). In the same way, if you find that you haven't practiced for a while, rather than criticizing yourself or ruminating about why, just *begin again, right there and then, by taking a 3-minute breathing space.*

2. Everyday Informal Mindfulness Practice

Lexy: *"Everyday mindfulness is a fantastic concept. I simply go about my tasks and activities for the day as normal, but choose to do them mindfully."*

In itself, mindfulness is not difficult—the challenge in everyday life is **remembering** to be mindful.

So, how can I best help myself remember to be mindful from hour to hour, day to day?

As best you can, hold the intention to be mindful lightly, rather than as yet another thing you "have" to do.

You might find it helpful to put reminder red dots or sticky notes in places where you will notice them (such as on your phone) or to download a mindfulness bell that sounds on your computer or smart phone during the day to invite you to reconnect with the here and now, or take a breathing space (see Resources).

Meditation teacher Larry Rosenberg offers these Five Reminders for Practicing Mindfulness throughout the Day:

1. When possible, do just one thing at a time.
2. Pay full attention to what you are doing.
3. When your mind wanders from what you are doing, bring it back.
4. Repeat step number three several billion times.
5. Investigate your distractions.

You might also find it helpful to revisit these practices from time to time as a reminder of some other possibilities for everyday informal mindfulness:

Bringing Awareness to Routine Activities Week 1, pages 55–57; Week 2, pages 76–77.

Pleasant Experiences Calendar, pages 77–81.

Unpleasant Experiences Calendar, pages 101–105.

Staying Present, page 185.

Mindful Walking, pages 125–128.

Some Tips for Everyday Mindfulness

- When you first wake up in the morning, before you get out of bed, bring your attention to your breathing. Observe five mindful breaths.

- Notice changes in your posture. Be aware of how your body and mind feel when you move from lying down to sitting, to standing, to walking. Notice each time you make a transition from one posture to the next.

- Whenever you hear a phone ring, a bird sing, a train pass by, laughter, a car horn, the wind, the sound of a door closing—use any sound as the bell of mindfulness. Really listen and be present and awake.

- Throughout the day, take a few moments to bring your attention to your breathing. Observe five mindful breaths.

- Whenever you eat or drink something, take a minute and breathe. Look at your food and realize that the food was connected to something that nourished its growth. Can you see the sunlight, the rain, the earth, the farmer, the trucker in your food? Pay attention as you eat, consciously consuming this food for your physical health. Bring awareness to seeing your food, smelling your food, tasting your food, chewing your food, and swallowing your food.

- Notice your body while you walk or stand. Take a moment to notice your posture. Pay attention to the contact of your feet with the ground under them. Feel the air on your face, arms, and legs as you walk. Are you rushing?

- Bring awareness to listening and talking. Can you listen without agreeing or disagreeing, liking or disliking, or planning what you will say when it is your turn? When talking, can you just say what you need to say without overstating or understating? Can you notice how your mind and body feel?

- Whenever you wait in a line, use this time to notice standing and breathing. Feel the contact of your feet with the floor and how your body feels. Bring attention to the rise and fall of your abdomen. Are you feeling impatient?

- Be aware of any points of tightness in your body throughout the day. See if you can breathe into them and, as you exhale, let go of excess tension. Is tension stored anywhere in your body? For example, your neck, shoulders, stomach, jaw, or lower back? If possible, stretch or do yoga once a day.

- Focus attention on your daily activities such as brushing your teeth, washing up, brushing your hair, putting on your shoes, doing your job. Bring mindfulness to each activity.

- Before you go to sleep at night, take a few minutes and bring your attention to your breathing. Observe five mindful breaths.

MADELINE KLYNE

3. The 3-Minute Breathing Space—Responsive

The breathing space is the single most important practice
in the whole MBCT program:
It's your way to switch into being mode
when you most need to do so.

Let it be your first response whenever you become aware that you are becoming entangled in unpleasant feelings, confused, unbalanced, or preoccupied.

To keep this vital practice fully alive and available, we suggest you **take at least one responsive breathing space** *every day*—life being as it is, you will probably not be short of opportunities for practice! Here's a reminder of the key steps (to show the importance of setting up your posture we've called this Step 0):

The Responsive Breathing Space

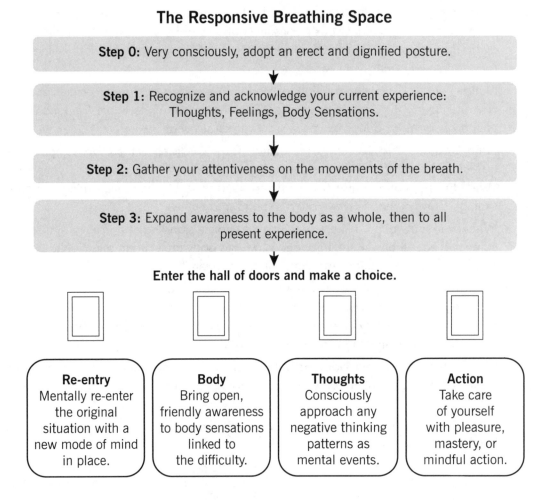

Step 0: Very consciously, adopt an erect and dignified posture.

Step 1: Recognize and acknowledge your current experience: Thoughts, Feelings, Body Sensations.

Step 2: Gather your attentiveness on the movements of the breath.

Step 3: Expand awareness to the body as a whole, then to all present experience.

Enter the hall of doors and make a choice.

Re-entry	**Body**	**Thoughts**	**Action**
Mentally re-enter the original situation with a new mode of mind in place.	Bring open, friendly awareness to body sensations linked to the difficulty.	Consciously approach any negative thinking patterns as mental events.	Take care of yourself with pleasure, mastery, or mindful action.

As We Close

We have come to the end of this part of our journey.

The practice of mindfulness offers, if we choose to take it, a continuing path forward—a path of discovery that can reveal entirely new ways of being in the world, ways that until now have remained, for many of us, largely unexplored and unexperienced.

We may discover that it is possible, strange as it may seem, to befriend ourselves as we are, right now, rather than striving to be someone else or somewhere else.

We may see that, once the harsh inner critic has been acknowledged, its insistent shout is not the only voice there is; that there is also a quieter, wiser, and more discerning voice that sees more clearly, and more kindly, what is to be done, even in the most difficult of situations.

Meditation is not about distancing ourselves from life and from our emotions. It is about truly participating, so that we are able to live authentically, to feel deeply and to act compassionately.

We can all so easily become strangers to ourselves.

Mindfulness offers a way home.

We wish you well as you continue your own unique journey of discovery day by day and moment by moment.

Love after Love

The time will come
when, with elation
you will greet yourself arriving
at your own door, in your own mirror
and each will smile at the other's welcome,

and say, sit here. Eat.
You will love again the stranger who was your self.
Give wine. Give bread. Give back your heart
to itself, to the stranger who has loved you

all your life, whom you ignored
for another, who knows you by heart.
Take down the love letters from the bookshelf,

the photographs, the desperate notes,
peel your own image from the mirror.
Sit. Feast on your life.

DEREK WALCOTT

Resources

Finding an MBCT Group

If you are not already participating in an MBCT group, but would like to explore the possibility of joining one, the easiest way is to search the Internet.

You can do this with Google or another search engine using a search string such as [mindfulness-based cognitive therapy + "your location"], or [mindfulness-based stress reduction + "your location"] or [mindfulness therapy + "your location"].

This should turn up leads on local mindfulness resources in your community. You can then ask more specifically about MBCT groups.

There are also a number of websites that list MBCT instructors offering groups in particular cities around the world. Some can be found under the "Resources" tab at *www.mbct.com/Resources_Main.htm*. For the United Kingdom, you can browse the "Find a Course near You" on *www.bemindful.co.uk*.

You might like to know that you can also take the MBCT course online at *www.bemindfulonline.com*.

Further Reading

More on Mindfulness-Based Programs

Kabat-Zinn, J. *Full Catastrophe Living: Using the Wisdom of Your Body and Mind to Face Stress, Pain and Illness, Second Edition.* New York: Bantam Books Trade Paperbacks, 2013.

This is a revised and updated edition of the original, classic text, first describing the Mindfulness-Based Stress Reduction (MBSR) program, on which mindfulness-based cognitive therapy is based.

Williams, J. M. G., Segal, Z. V., Teasdale, J. D., & Kabat-Zinn, J. *The Mindful Way through Depression: Freeing Yourself from Chronic Unhappiness.* New York: Guilford Press, 2007.

This offers an extended narrative description of the background, ideas, practices, and effects of the MBCT in depression program. It includes guided meditations narrated by Jon Kabat-Zinn.

Orsillo, S., & Roemer, E. *The Mindful Way through Anxiety.* New York: Guilford Press, 2011.

This book uses a similar format to *The Mindful Way through Depression* and is specifically written for people suffering from disturbing fears and anxiety who want to learn how the integration of traditional exposure techniques with mindfulness training can help them live more fully.

Germer, C. *The Mindful Path to Self-Compassion.* New York: Guilford Press, 2007.

This book offers helpful guidance in addressing self-blame, judgment, and perfectionism through developing mindfulness and compassionate responses to difficulties.

Williams, M., & Penman, D. *Mindfulness: A Practical Guide to Finding Peace in a Frantic World.* London: Piatkus, 2011.

This general book, based on *The Mindful Way through Depression*, describes how the practice of mindfulness can be broadened to deal with milder, common mental states such as worry and unhappiness. It is focused on cultivating a sense of peace and wellness in the midst of the busyness of ordinary life. It includes downloads of shorter meditations, narrated by Mark Williams; see *www.franticworld.com*).

The MBCT Manual

Segal, Z. V., Williams, J. M. G., & Teasdale, J. D. *Mindfulness-Based Cognitive Therapy for Depression, Second Edition.* New York: Guilford Press, 2013.

This is the full manual that health professionals use as the basis of MBCT teaching—in case you want to go really deeply into the history, ideas, practices, research, and teaching of the program.

More on Mindfulness

Kabat-Zinn, J. *Wherever You Go, There You Are: Mindfulness Meditation in Everyday Life.* New York: Hyperion Press, 1994.

Kabat-Zinn, J. *Coming to Our Senses: Healing Ourselves and the World Through Mindfulness.* New York: Hyperion Press, 2005.

Hanh, T. N. *The Miracle of Mindfulness.* Boston: Beacon Press, 1976.

Henepola, G. *Mindfulness in Plain English.* Somerville, MA: Wisdom Publications, 1992.

See also *www.oxfordmindfulness.org*, *www.mbct.com*, and *www.bemindful.co.uk*.

Acceptance and Kindness

Brach, T. *Radical Acceptance*. New York: Bantam Books, 2004.

Salzberg, S. *Lovingkindness: The Revolutionary Art of Happiness*. Boston: Shambhala Publications, 1995.

The Practice of Insight Meditation

Mindfulness-based applications (such as MBSR and MBCT) are closely related to the Westernized insight meditation tradition. This approach to meditation is not focused on particular emotional disorders but aims to reduce suffering and enhance freedom of heart and mind more generally.

The book *Seeking the Heart of Wisdom*, by Joseph Goldstein and Jack Kornfield (Boston: Shambhala Publications, 2001), offers a fine introductory description.

If you would like to explore practicing this approach on your own, we recommend:

Goldstein, J., & Salzberg, S. *Insight Meditation Kit: A Step by Step Course on How to Meditate*. Louisville, CO: Sounds True Audio, 2002.

If you wish to explore this approach more deeply, it is best to get teaching directly from a meditation teacher experienced in this tradition. A number of centers offer this possibility. See the following for further details.

In North America:

Insight Meditation Society in Barre, Massachusetts
www.dharma.org

Spirit Rock in Woodacre, California
www.spiritrock.org

In Europe:

Gaia House in Devon, England
www.gaiahouse.co.uk

In Australia:

Australian Insight Meditation Network
www.dharma.org.au

Additional Websites Offering Resources on Mindfulness

www.oxfordmindfulness.org
Website of the University of Oxford Mindfulness Centre, with links to other U.K.

universities that teach mindfulness (for example, Bangor, Exeter) and links to many other resources (such as guided meditations and podcasts) to help you.

www.stressreductiontapes.com
For tapes/CDs of meditation practices recorded by Jon Kabat-Zinn.

www.mindfulnessdc.org/bell/index.html
A website that allows you to set a bell as a reminder to be mindful throughout your day.

www.umassmed.edu/cfm
Website of the Center for Mindfulness, University of Massachusetts Medical School.

www.mentalhealth.org.uk
Mental Health Foundation: report on MBCT; access to material on mindfulness under "Be Mindful" and "Wellbeing podcasts."

Notes

Chapter 1: Welcome

Page 3

MBCT has been tested in research and proven effective for depression, as well as for anxiety and a range of other problems: Drawing on six randomized trials of 593 patients, a meta-analysis conducted by J. Piet and E. Hougaard (The effect of mindfulness-based cognitive therapy for prevention of relapse in recurrent major depression: A systematic review and meta-analysis, *Clinical Psychology Review* 2011; *31:* 1032–1040) reported that MBCT significantly reduced the risk of relapse, relative to staying with usual care, by 43% for participants with three or more past episodes of depression. They also reported that MBCT and antidepressant medication reduced relapse risk to a similar degree.

In a second meta-analysis, S. G. Hofman and colleagues (The effect of mindfulness-based therapy on anxiety and depression: A meta-analytic review, *Journal of Consulting and Clinical Psychology* 2010; *78:* 169–183) scrutinized 1,140 patients receiving mindfulness-based interventions for a variety of mental health conditions and examined reductions in symptoms of anxiety and depression, rather than whether a person relapsed or not. Treatments featuring mindfulness training, of which MBCT is a prominent example, had large and similar effect sizes for both anxious and depressive symptoms. These benefits were maintained past the point at which patients were no longer receiving treatment.

Perhaps the most compelling endorsement for MBCT comes from the United Kingdom's National Institute for Health and Care Excellence (NICE), an independent national body that provides clinical guidelines for evidence-based care to patients using the National Health Service. Guidelines are formulated through a stringent review of empirical and clinical studies for a particular medical or psychiatric condition and recommendations reflect the most supported treatments. The NICE guidelines for unipolar depression have, since 2004, consistently endorsed MBCT as an effective means for prevention of relapse and recurrence.

Page 4

MBCT Is Effective. See note for Chapter 1, page 3.

Page 5

two critical processes that lie at the root of depression and many other emotional problems: 1. the tendency to overthink, ruminate, or worry too much about some things, *coupled with* 2. a tendency to avoid, suppress, or push away other things. For the tendency to overthink, ruminate, etc., see Nolen-Hoeksema, S., *Overthinking: Women Who Think Too Much.* New York: Holt, 2002. For the tendency to avoid, etc., see Hayes, S. C., and colleagues, Experiential avoidance and behavioural disorders: A functional dimensional approach to diagnosis and treatment. *Journal of Consulting and Clinical Psychology,* 1996, *64,* 1152–1168.

Page 6

Research is constantly expanding the range of emotional problems that benefit from MBCT. See page 407 in Segal, Z. V., Williams, J. M. G., and Teasdale, J. D., *Mindfulness-Based Cognitive Therapy for Depression: A New Approach to Preventing Relapse, Second Edition.* New York: Guilford Press, 2013.

Page 7

There is also growing evidence that MBCT can help people while they are in the midst of a depression. See, for example, J. R. van Aalderen and colleagues, The efficacy of mindfulness-based cognitive therapy in recurrent depressed patients with and without a current depressive episode: A randomized controlled trial. *Psychological Medicine,* 2012, *42,* 989–1001.

The patterns of mind. Teasdale, J. D., and Chaskalson, M. How does mindfulness transform suffering? I: The nature and origins of *dukkha. Contemporary Buddhism: An Interdisciplinary Journal,* 2011, *12* (1), 89–102. Copyright 2011 by Taylor and Francis.

The Mindful Way through Depression was written by Mark Williams, John Teasdale, Zindel Segal, and Jon Kabat-Zinn and was published in 2007 by The Guilford Press, New York.

Chapter 2: Depression, Unhappiness, and Emotional Distress: Why Do We Get Stuck?

Page 12

Research using this list of words has revealed something very important. Teasdale, J. D., and Cox, S. G. Dysphoria: Self-devaluative and affective components in recovered depressed patients and never depressed controls. *Psychological Medicine,* 2001, *31,* 1311–1316.

Page 13

Moods and feelings can trigger "matching" patterns of thinking, memory, and attention. See, for example, Fox, E., *Emotion Science: Neuroscientific and Cognitive Approaches to Understanding Human Emotions*. Basingstoke, U.K.: Palgrave Macmillan, 2008.

Page 15

Ruminating just makes us feel even worse. See Nolen-Hoeksema, S., *Overthinking: Women Who Think Too Much*. New York: Holt, 2002.

Chapter 3. Doing, Being, and Mindfulness

Page 21

Being and doing were first discussed in relation to mindfulness-based applications by Jon Kabat-Zinn in his 1990 book *Full Catastrophe Living: Using the Wisdom of Your Body and Mind to Face Stress, Pain and Illness* (New York: Dell), and then further elaborated as modes of mind in relation to MBCT in Zindel Segal, Mark Williams, and John Teasdale's 2002 book *Mindfulness-Based Cognitive Therapy for Depression: A New Approach to Preventing Relapse* (New York: Guilford Press) and in Mark Williams, John Teasdale, Zindel Segal, and Jon Kabat-Zinn's 2007 work *The Mindful Way through Depression* (New York: Guilford Press).

Page 26

Mindfulness is the awareness that emerges through paying attention in a particular way: on purpose, in the present moment, and nonjudgmentally to things as they are. This is based on Jon Kabat-Zinn's description on page 4 in *Wherever You Go There You Are: Mindfulness Meditation in Everyday Life*. New York: Hyperion, 1994.

"The quality of mindfulness is not a neutral or blank presence. True mindfulness is imbued with warmth, compassion, and interest." Feldman, C., *The Buddhist Path to Simplicity,* page 173. London: Thorsons, 2001.

Page 29

MBCT works by teaching us to be more mindful, kinder, and more compassionate. See Kuyken, W., and colleagues, How does mindfulness-based cognitive therapy work? *Behaviour Research and Therapy*, 2010, *48*, 1105–1112.

Page 30

MBCT: A Brief History. See the note for Chapter 1, page 3.

Chapter 5. Week 1: Beyond Automatic Pilot

Page 40

If I Had My Life to Live Over. The origins of this piece attributed to Nadine Stair are obscure.

Page 42

An Eating Meditation. Based on Kabat-Zinn, J., *Full Catastrophe Living,* pages 27–28. New York: Dell, 1990.

Page 47

Body Scan Meditation. From Williams, J. M. G., Teasdale, J. D., Segal, Z. V., and Kabat-Zinn, J., *The Mindful Way through Depression.* New York: Guilford Press, 2007. Copyright 2007 by The Guilford Press. Adapted by permission.

Page 55

Looking Back. From Segal, Z. V., Williams, J. M. G., and Teasdale, J. D., *Mindfulness-Based Cognitive Therapy for Depression, Second Edition.* New York: Guilford Press, 2013. Copyright 2013 by The Guilford Press.

Page 59

You Reading This, Be Ready. From Stafford, W. E., *The Way It Is: New and Selected Poems.* Minneapolis: Graywolf Press, 1998. Copyright 1998 by the Estate of William Stafford. Reprinted by permission of The Permissions Company, Inc., on behalf of Graywolf Press, Minneapolis, MN, *www.graywolfpress.org.*

Chapter 6. Week 2: Another Way of Knowing

Page 66

Our moods affect how we interpret events in ways that keep the moods going. See, for example, Fox, E., *Emotion Science: Neuroscientific and Cognitive Approaches to Understanding Human Emotions.* Basingstoke, U. K.: Palgrave Macmillan, 2008.

Page 73

10-Minute Mindfulness of Breathing Meditation. Adapted from Segal, Z. V., Williams, J. M. G., and Teasdale, J. D., *Mindfulness-Based Cognitive Therapy for Depression, Second Edition.* New York: Guilford Press, 2013. Copyright 2013 by The Guilford Press. Adapted by permission.

Page 82

Dreaming the Real. From France, L., Dreaming the Real, in Abhinando Bhikkhu (Ed.), *Tomorrow's Moon*. Harnham, Northumberland, UK: Aruna Publications, 2005. Copyright 2005 by Linda France. Reprinted by permission.

Chapter 7. Week 3: Coming Home to the Present— Gathering the Scattered Mind

Page 85

Stretch and Breath Meditation: Mindful Stretching. Adapted from Segal, Z. V., Williams, J. M. G., and Teasdale, J. D., *Mindfulness-Based Cognitive Therapy for Depression, Second Edition*. New York: Guilford Press, 2013. Copyright 2013 by The Guilford Press. Adapted by permission.

Page 98

3-Minute Breathing Space Instructions. Adapted from Williams, J. M. G., Teasdale, J. D., Segal, Z. V., and Kabat-Zinn, J., *The Mindful Way through Depression*. New York: Guilford Press, 2007. Copyright 2007 by The Guilford Press. Adapted by permission.

Page 106

The Peace of Wild Things. From Berry, W., *New Collected Poems*. Berkeley, CA: Counterpoint, 2012. Copyright 2012 by Wendell Berry. Reprinted by permission of Counterpoint.

Chapter 8. Week 4: Recognizing Aversion

Page 111

Checklist of Negative Thoughts. The questionnaire used here is an adapted version of the Automatic Thoughts Questionnaire from Hollon, S. D., and Kendall, P., Cognitive self-statements in depression: Development of an Automatic Thoughts Questionnaire. *Cognitive Therapy and Research,* 1980, *4,* 383–395. Copyright 1980 by Philip C. Kendall and Steven D. Hollon. Adapted by permission of the authors.

Page 115

Sitting Meditation: Mindfulness of Breath, Body, Sounds, Thoughts, and Choiceless Awareness. Adapted from Segal, Z. V., Williams, J. M. G., and Teasdale, J. D., *Mindfulness-Based Cognitive Therapy for Depression, Second Edition*. New York: Guilford Press, 2013. Copyright 2013 by The Guilford Press. Adapted by permission.

Page 126

Mindful Walking. Adapted from Segal, Z. V., Williams, J. M. G., and Teasdale, J. D., *Mindfulness-Based Cognitive Therapy for Depression, Second Edition.* New York: Guilford Press, 2013. Copyright 2013 by The Guilford Press. Adapted by permission.

Page 129

Wild Geese. From Oliver, M., *Dream Work.* Copyright 1986 by Mary Oliver. Reprinted by permission of Grove/Atlantic, Inc.

Chapter 9. Week 5: Allowing Things to Be as They Already Are

Page 132

The Guest House. From Barks, C., and Moyne, J., *The Essential Rumi.* New York: Harper Collins, 1995. Copyright 1995 by Coleman Barks and John Moyne. Originally published by Threshold Books. Reprinted by permission of Threshold Books.

Page 136

Inviting Difficulty In and Working with It through the Body. Adapted from Segal, Z. V., Williams, J. M. G., and Teasdale, J. D. *Mindfulness-Based Cognitive Therapy for Depression, Second Edition.* New York: Guilford Press, 2013. Copyright 2013 by The Guilford Press. Adapted by permission.

Page 142

Maria. Adapted from Segal, Z. V., Williams, J. M. G., and Teasdale, J. D. *Mindfulness-Based Cognitive Therapy for Depression, Second Edition,* pages 283–285. New York: Guilford Press, 2013. Copyright 2013 by The Guilford Press. Adapted by permission.

Page 144

Using the Breathing Space: Extra Guidance. Adapted from Segal, Z. V., Williams, J. M. G., and Teasdale, J. D. *Mindfulness-Based Cognitive Therapy for Depression, Second Edition.* New York: Guilford Press, 2013. Copyright 2013 by The Guilford Press. Adapted by permission.

Page 147

Prelude. From Dreamer, O. M., *The Dance.* New York: HarperCollins, 2001. Copyright 2001 by Oriah Mountain Dreamer. Reprinted by permission of HarperCollins Publishers.

Chapter 10. Week 6: Seeing Thoughts *as* Thoughts

Page 149

The Office. This exercise is adapted, with permission, from one devised by Isabel Hargreaves (personal communication, 1995).

Page 154

The Train of Associations. Adapted from Goldstein, J., *Insight Meditation: The Practice of Freedom,* pages 59–60. Boston: Shambhala, 1994. Copyright 1994 by Joseph Goldstein. Adapted by arrangement with Shambhala Publications, Inc., Boston, *www.shambhala.com.*

Page 160

"It is amazing to observe how much power we give unknowingly to uninvited thoughts." From Goldstein, J., *Insight Meditation: The Practice of Freedom,* page 60. Boston: Shambhala, 1994. Copyright 1994 by Joseph Goldstein. Reprinted by permission of Shambhala Publications, Inc., Boston, *www.shambhala.com.*

Page 169

Stepping Back from Thought. Adapted from Kabat-Zinn, J., *Full Catastrophe Living.* New York: Dell, 1990. Copyright 1990 by Jon Kabat-Zinn. Adapted by permission of Dell Publishing, a division of Random House, Inc.

Chapter 11. Week 7: Kindness in Action

Page 172

Research has revealed the encouraging truth that skillful use of activity, by itself, can be an effective treatment for depression. See, for example, Dobson, K. S., and colleagues, Randomized trial of behavioral activation, cognitive therapy, and antidepressant medication in the prevention of relapse and recurrence in major depression. *Journal of Consulting and Clinical Psychology,* 2008, 76, 468–477.

Page 178

Jackie. Adapted from Segal, Z. V., Williams, J. M. G., and Teasdale, J. D., *Mindfulness-Based Cognitive Therapy for Depression, Second Edition.* New York: Guilford Press, 2013. Copyright 2013 by The Guilford Press. Adapted by permission.

Page 183

The Breathing Space: The Door of Mindful Action. Adapted from Segal, Z. V., Williams, J. M. G., and Teasdale, J. D. *Mindfulness-Based Cognitive Therapy for Depression, Second Edition.* New York: Guilford Press, 2013. Copyright 2013 by The Guilford Press. Adapted by permission.

Page 185

Staying Present. Adapted from Goldstein, J., *Insight Meditation: The Practice of Freedom.* Boston: Shambhala, 1994. Copyright 1994 by Joseph Goldstein. Adapted by permission from Shambhala Publications, Inc., Boston, *www.shambhala.com.*

Page 195

The Summer Day. From Oliver, M., *House of Light.* Boston: Beacon Press, 1990. Copyright 1990 by Mary Oliver. Reprinted by permission of The Charlotte Sheedy Literary Agency, Inc.

Chapter 12. Week 8: What Now?

Page 205

Some Tips That Other Participants Found Helpful. Our thanks to our colleagues Becca Crane, Marie Johansson, Sarah Silverton, Christina Surawy, and Thorsten Barnhofer for sharing their participants' experiences.

Page 206

Meditation teacher Larry Rosenberg offers these Five Reminders for Practicing Mindfulness throughout the Day. From Rosenberg, L., *Breath by Breath: The Liberating Practice of Insight Meditation,* pages 168–170. Boston: Shambhala, 1998.

Page 207

Some Tips for Everyday Mindfulness. Adapted from an unpublished work by Madeline Klyne, Executive Director, Cambridge Insight Meditation Center. Copyright by Madeline Klyne. Adapted by permission.

Page 210

Love after Love. From Walcott, D., *Collected Poems, 1948–1984.* New York: Farrar, Straus and Giroux, 1986. Copyright 1986 by Derek Walcott. Reprinted by permission of Farrar, Straus and Giroux, LLC, and Faber and Faber Ltd.

Index

About the Authors

John Teasdale, PhD, held a Special Scientific Appointment with the United Kingdom Medical Research Council's Cognition and Brain Sciences Unit in Cambridge. He is a Fellow of the British Academy and the Academy of Medical Sciences. He collaborated with Mark Williams and Zindel Segal in developing mindfulness-based cognitive therapy (MBCT) to prevent relapse and recurrence in major depression; together, they coauthored *Mindfulness-Based Cognitive Therapy for Depression, Second Edition* (for mental health professionals), as well as (with Jon Kabat-Zinn) the self-help guide *The Mindful Way through Depression*. Since retiring, Dr. Teasdale has taught mindfulness and insight meditation internationally. He continues to explore and seek to understand the wider implications of mindfulness and meditation for enhancing our way of being.

Mark Williams, DPhil, is Professor of Clinical Psychology Emeritus and Honorary Senior Research Fellow at the University of Oxford Department of Psychiatry, where he was Founding Director of the Oxford Mindfulness Centre. In addition to his books with John Teasdale et al., Dr. Williams is coauthor of *Mindfulness-Based Cognitive Therapy with People at Risk for Suicide* (for mental health professionals). He continues to work with colleagues to research the role of mindfulness in the prevention of depression in adolescents, and to train new mindfulness teachers internationally. He is a Fellow of the Academy of Medical Sciences and the British Academy.

Zindel Segal, PhD, is Distinguished Professor of Psychology in Mood Disorders at the University of Toronto–Scarborough. He is Director of Clinical Training in the Clinical Psychological Science Program and is also Professor in the Department of Psychiatry. Dr. Segal has conducted influential research into the psychological processes that make certain people more vulnerable than others to developing depression and experiencing recurrent episodes. He actively advocates for the relevance of mindfulness-based clinical care in psychiatry and mental health.

List of Audio Files

	Track Title	Run Time	Voice
1	Welcome	00:31	John Teasdale
2	Raisin Exercise	09:53	Zindel Segal
3	Body Scan	39:08	John Teasdale
4	10-Minute Sitting Meditation—Mindfulness of the Breath	09:54	Mark Williams
5	Mindful Movement—Formal Practice	38:30	Zindel Segal
6	Stretch and Breath Meditation	33:39	Mark Williams
7	Mindful Walking	13:42	Mark Williams
8	3-Minute Breathing Space	05:02	John Teasdale
9	3-Minute Breathing Space—Extended Version	05:19	Zindel Segal
10	20-Minute Sitting Meditation	20:38	Zindel Segal
11	Sitting Meditation	37:47	John Teasdale
12	Working with Difficulty Meditation	25:47	Mark Williams
13	Bells at 5 Minutes, 10 Minutes, 15 Minutes, 20 Minutes, and 30 Minutes	30:10	
14	Two Ways of Knowing	07:06	John Teasdale

How to Listen to the MP3 CD

You can listen to the MP3 CD in many ways. If you have an MP3-enabled CD player (look for an MP3 logo on the device), you can play this disc just like any audio CD. You can play it on most computers by simply inserting it into the CD tray. You can also then copy the files onto an MP3 player or import the files into your iTunes library and listen on the go. The tracks are also available to download from The Guilford Press website, *www.guilford.com/teasdale-materials*.